THE HEALING POWER OF HYPNOTISM

Explains the true nature of hypnotism and the valuable part that it can play in modern medicine both in dealing with those suffering from emotional and neurotic problems and in helping healthy people to achieve a particular personal goal.

The Healing Power of HYPNOTISM

What It Is and How It Works

by

Caroline Shreeve
M.B., B.S.(Lond.), L.R.C.P., M.R.C.S.(Eng.)

and

David Shreeve
B.A.(Hons.), L.N.C.P.

Series Editor
George T. Lewith
M.A., M.R.C.G.P., M.R.C.P.

THORSONS

THORSONS PUBLISHERS LIMITED
Wellingborough, Northamptonshire

First published 1984
Second Impression 1985

British Library Cataloguing in Publication Data

Shreeve, Caroline
    The healing power of hypnotism
    1. Hypnotism — Therapeutic use
    I. Title   II. Shreeve, David
    615.8'512   RC495

ISBN 0-7225-0871-9

Printed and bound in Great Britain

We should like to dedicate this book to Norman Lee, President of the National Council of Psychotherapists, and to John Beard, secretary of the Council, in grateful recognition of their teaching, to which we owe whatever insight we possess into the healing art of hypnotherapy.

Contents

Foreword

Hypnotism, or animal magnetism as it was known when it was popularized by Mesmer in the eighteenth century, has been the subject of much debate. In some people's minds, particularly until this century, it was assumed to be complete shamanism. Hypnosis was somehow evil, almost equivalent to witchcraft, and certainly not a therapy to be promoted by the respectable element of the medical profession! Fortunately ideas and attitudes change, both because of innovative discoveries and in response to public demand.

Hypnotism, quite rightly, has become respectable. It has a proven effect and is certainly of enormous potential value to the practising physician. It can be used as a therapy in two main ways; either as an end in itself to modify or alter symptomatology (such as the desire to smoke) or as an investigative and therapeutic technique in psychotherapy.

There are probably more hypnotists now in the United Kingdom than there have ever been in the past, and the therapeutic value of hypnotism seems no longer to be in debate. Caroline Shreeve's book provides a clear exposition and allows the critical and objective reader to form a valid opinion about hypnosis and its potential value.

GEORGE T. LEWITH
M.A., M.R.C.P., M.R.C.G.P.
Southampton 1984

Introduction

The subject of hypnotism has always been — and may well remain for some time — a controversial one. But much work and intensive research has been carried out into this discipline over the past forty years, that it is becoming more and more firmly established as a valuable adjunct to traditional methods of diagnosing and treating psychological illness. In addition to this, of course, hypnotic techniques are extensively used to relieve or overcome a number of physical illnesses, and to eliminate unwanted social habits such as smoking, overeating, and addiction to alcohol. Over the past twenty-five years, in fact, hypnotherapy has gained familiarity and at the same time respectability with many members of the medical profession, who either learn to practise the art themselves or willingly refer appropriate patients to a qualified hypnotist. And as the number of hypnotherapists grows, many patients on their own initiative turn to them in the hope that they may help to solve mental or physical problems which have not responded to orthodox treatment.

Since we have become better informed, thanks to improved communications, education, coverage of research developments by the media etc., it is now a widely known fact that many physical ills have a largely psychological cause. Many asthmatic patients, for instance, tire of annual desensitization injections against a range of possible allergies or their propensity to have attacks of their illness at unpremeditated intervals, and consult a hypnotherapist rather than remain on a multiplicity of drugs.

And for asthma patients you may substitute chronic or acute arthritics; sufferers from acute or chronic pain of whatever origin; victims of abdominal, intestinal or gastric problems; women with period pain, infertility or frigidity; men with impotence or other sexual problems; and sufferers from high blood pressure, palpitations, mock angina, and recurrent housemaid's knee!

There is, in fact, no complaint which has not at some time been presented, advisedly or otherwise, to a hypnotherapist or inducer of trances, in either desperation or defiance at orthodox medicine's inability to heal, or at least relieve, its troublesome symptoms.

Hypnotherapy has not been the only form of alternative medicine to take root and flourish in our society over the past twenty years. Together with the New Age concept of a return to the earth and a simpler form of life, to gain inner awareness and peace and to avoid the stress and madness of the urban rat race, there has been a consistent tendency to re-examine ancient but unforgotten healing arts. This has been due to a renewed appreciation of the artistic or intuitive as opposed to the purely scientific aspects of medicine. I am not implying for a moment that the forms of alternative medicine referred to, such as acupuncture, naturopathy, osteopathy, chiropractice, herbalism etc. — let alone hypnotherapy — have no valid foundation. All of the healing arts 'work', i.e., succeed, in the hands of some of their practitioners upon some patients even though a number of them, such as homoeopathy, do not in fact withstand scrutiny in the light of established scientific fact. But while hypnotherapy shares with some of the other forms of alternative medicine the necessity for suitable temperament and an acquired judgement and skill (that is, artistic rather than scientific qualities of medical practice) so it may also justifiably be termed a science in that there is a demonstrable and repeatable relationship between cause and effect. And the hypnotic trance — the medium through which the therapist works — is accurately measurable in duration and depth.

Whether the hypnotherapeutic treatment is being carried out by a lay hypnotherapist or a doctor of medicine who has trained in the discipline himself, the increasing acceptance of hypnotism as a valid medical aid is turning the tables in the opposite direction to the way they were facing prior to the First World War and for intervals long preceding that.

Hypnotism was seen then to be able to cure various illnesses, but many bandwagon jumpers, get-rich-fast merchants and fraudulent quacks learned and misused the art for the purposes of showmanship and to earn a great deal of money for themselves. And this, together with the impressively 'magical' appearance of the actual art of hypnotizing a subject, made orthodox medical practitioners highly sceptical of the art and highly condemnatory of it. This left the public to fall between two stools. Either they accepted the limitations of orthodox medical treatment and scorned or pretended to scorn the mysteries of hypnotism, or they fell prey to the impressive acts often available as entertainment by eager stage hypnotists and ran the risk of a fleecing if they happened to approach an unethical therapist about their illness or complaint.

Nowadays the establishment of hypnotherapy as practised by lay and medically qualified therapists has integrated it firmly as an adjunct rather than as an alternative to routine medical practice, and patients by and large can expect to have a sympathetic hearing if they request their GP to recommend a local hypnotherapist.

Some people today associate the name 'hypnotism' with the older name of Mesmerism and believe that the art came into being as a result of Franz Mesmer's work and writings during the eighteenth century. So it is interesting to know that the origins of hypnotism lay shrouded in the mists of antiquity, for healing in a trance state is one of the oldest of the medical arts. Primitive man is known to have practised it and he attributed a divine origin to the trance state, ascribing miraculous cures to the benevolent attitudes of the tribal gods. The Ebers papyrus, which is over 3000 years old, describes the hypnotic procedures used by Egyptian soothsayers and these have a lot in common with current hypnotic practice. The Hindu fakirs, the Persian magi, the Indian yogi and the Greek oracles also used similar methods under different names, and the earliest medical records describe miraculous healing by priests whose ritual magic brought about trance-like conditions in worshippers in the Aesculapian temples.

Belief in miraculous cures persisted into the Middle Ages and it was thought that health could be brought about in diseased or crippled people through contact with the water of healing springs and wells, religious statues or holy relics. The power of suggestion can also be seen at work in the effecting of miracle cures by kings and religious leaders. Both English and French monarchs were thought to possess the power to 'lay on hands' and heal the sick, the practice being known as 'touching for the King's evil'. It seems likely that 'cures' as far apart in time as the biblical miracle cures and those that occur annually at Fatima and Lourdes, are equally valid examples of the power of suggestibility.

At least until 1530, no explanation beyond divine intervention was sought for phenomena effected in trance states which we today recognize as being hypnotic in character. In that year, Paracelsus, a scientist and physician of Swiss origin whose real name was Philipp Theophrastus Bombast von Hohenheim, evolved his theory about the interrelationship between the stars and man, especially about the effect of the former upon human disease processes. This is one of the origins of medical astrology as it is known today and from it developed the idea that not only did stars and planets influence men but also that men and women can influence one another through the medium of magnetic power.

The next historical figure to have comparable views on 'animal magnetism' and to make his mark on history because of his work on the subject, was Franz Anton Mesmer (1734-1815). He was an Austrian physician to whom much is attributed but whose theories and writings have recently been shown to have plagiarized the original work of the brilliant English physician, Richard Mead (1673-1754). Mead had been directly inspired by the research of his patient, Sir Isaac Newton. From work carried out by Richard Mead, Mesmer later developed his 'universal fluid' idea. This fluid he considered to be the medium through which planets influence human health, and thought of it as a transparent and odourless gass in which all bodies are immersed. He started treating patients by means of magnets applied to the painful or diseased areas of their bodies to which the magnets were carefully moulded, at the same time investigating the properties of magnetic force.

Mesmer's surprising and dramatic cures attracted a great deal of fame and at the same time aroused sufficient antagonism among his medical colleagues to oblige him to leave Vienna where he was then working. He went to live in Paris and there he founded one of the most famous of European medical clinics. When treating patients he employed elaborate apparatus and ceremonial ritual comparable in style and magnificence to that generally used at religious shrines. We have a good description of the scenes of healing in Mesmer's inimitable fashion. The patients were shown into a large, thickly curtained, dark room to the accompaniment of appropriate piano music to set the atmosphere.

A large oak tub — the famous 'baquet' — stood in the middle of the room containing a mixture of water, powdered glass and iron filings.

This was covered by a perforated lid and emerging through the holes were jointed iron rods. The patients, in strictly observed silence, joined hands and applied the projecting rods to the diseased parts of their bodies. This was the point at which the great master, Mesmer, appeared. He wore a pale lilac, silk robe and held a long iron wand in his hand. He passed slowly and gravely among the patients, watching them and touching them here and there with his hands or the tip of his iron wand. Some patients remained unaffected by these ministrations, but others were rapidly overcome by paroxysms of spitting and coughing, and experienced a sensation of insects running over their skins. A few, particularly excitable and nervous young ladies, would fall down in a fit and convulse on the floor at Mesmer's very feet.

These various physical reactions among the patients were known as the 'crisis' and augured well for the ultimate recovery from whatever was afflicting them. Two or three sessions of this type cured a very large number of people of a vast variety of disorders, and Mesmer's fame spread far and wide.

Certainly his treatment was based on false premises. Believing that planets could effect change in the human body through the medium of the invisible magnetic fluid, he also thought that the human will could activate the fluid, withdrawing it from one place and getting it to accumulate at another, thereby producing surprising results. He named the fluid 'animal magnetism' and attributed disease to an unbalanced distribution of this fluid in the patient's body. When he passed his wand or hand over various areas of the sick person, Mesmer maintained that invisible magnetic fluid flowed out through the tips of his fingers or the end of the rod, into the patient's body, redistributing the fluid and thereby restoring harmony. This successfully gave rise to renewed health.

False premises apart, Mesmer doubtless cured a large number of so-called incurable people and in so doing, angered his medical colleagues a great deal. In 1784, Louis XVI appointed a committee to investigate the matter, at the request of the leading members of the Paris medical profession. Mesmerism, or animal magnetism as it was then called, was discredited as no foundation for it could be discovered. The final crushing verdict was that imagination and imitation were the only real forces at work and that ultimately the effects of treatment would be bound to be harmful.

The committee's report ruined Mesmer's reputation and fashion turned against him. This was very sad — from several points of view. Regardless of the underlying false notions, there is no doubt that people genuinely benefitted from the treatment and were very unlikely despite the committee's feelings on the matter to have been harmed in any way from it. It either left them as they were, or relieved them of illness, and that is more than can be claimed for many of the forms of orthodox treatment available today. In addition, Mesmer, however much he loved an impressive display, sincerely believed the ideas he propounded and wished to cure people of their sickness. The medical profession hated him because he could cure people whom they had failed to cure — and thereby acquire fame, popularity and money. It is no wonder that their prejudice against Mesmerism knew no bounds!

The next important development in the history of animal magnetism as it was still called, occurred in 1787, three years after the findings of the committee that ended Mesmer's Parisian fame. The Marquis de Puységur, one of Mesmer's disciples, described a condition later known as artificial somnambulism. This was a kind of sleep in which the magnetizer could direct the ideas and actions of the magnetized subject. Later, at the beginning of the nineteenth century, Bertrand attributed this state entirely to the workings of the subject's imagination. This significant finding was utilized effectively by the Abbé Faria, the first recorded person to induce the state simply by saying to his subjects: 'I wish you to go to sleep!' But the continuous antagonism of the medical profession forced the development of Mesmerism to a standstill for over sixty years.

During this time the art was exploited by conjurors and show businessmen at travelling fairs, who used it to demonstrate trance phenomena to amazed audiences. In 1841, a well-known Manchester surgeon named James Braid, watched a demonstration of magnetic experiments, and finding trance induction to be perfectly genuine, started to experiment himself. On obtaining excellent results in both medical and surgical cases, he offered in 1842 to read a paper he had written on the subject to the British Association for the Advancement of Science. But his offer was rejected and his paper denigrated as ridiculous.

Several years later the physician Elliotson was dismissed from his professorial post at University College, London, simply because he chose hypnotism as the subject for his Harveian oration. At about this time, James Esdale, who was practising surgery in India, sent a report to the medical board of seventy-five operations which he had performed painlessly under hypnotic anaesthesia; but his letter was never even acknowledged.

All three men, Braid, Elliotson and Esdale are remarkable in that they, as doctors, became convinced of the validity of hypnotic trance induction but were unable to effect any change in the attitude of their colleagues. James Braid is particularly memorable, because apart from conducting experiments himself into trance phenomena and putting his findings to use in treating both medical and surgical cases, he also advanced the idea that far from being due to an invisible magnetic fluid, results obtained under hypnosis were purely subjective in nature. 'The phenomena', he said, 'are due to suggestion alone, acting upon a subject whose suggestibility has been artificially increased.'

This marks the beginning of the discovery of the equation representing the induction of hypnosis, namely:

Misdirected attention + belief + expectation + imagination = the hypnotic state.

This equation applies for all time and regardless of the form in which hypnotic trance is manifesting itself, be it trance induction by a hypnotist, faith healing, or miraculous cures occurring at a holy shrine or well. No psychological cures have ever taken place in the absence of belief and we owe the invention of the word 'hypnotism' to James Braid who regarded the trance as similar to the sleeping state (Hypnos was the Greek god of sleep). Forthwith the names Mesmerism and 'animal magnetism' were used less and less.

The father of modern hypnotism can really be considered to be Ambroise Auguste Liébault of Nancy, France. His book Le Sommeil Provoqué (Induced Sleep) was published in 1889, and he founded the practice of the therapeutics of suggestion. He was indubitably the first person to demonstrate the healing power of hypnotism on a large scale, treating thousands of people successfully by his methods. Professor Bernheim, a famous and accomplished neurologist also from Nancy, soon heard about

Liébault's work, and was so incensed by stories of cures he considered must be pure trickery that he decided to visit Liébault's clinic and expose the physician as a fraudulent quack.

However, he was so surprised and impressed by all that he saw, that he was rapidly converted to Liébault's views and, in turn, became one of the leading authorities on the subject. His renown as a physician throughout Europe was such that for the first time ever, the medical profession was unable to ignore the findings of hypnosis and maintain its hostile attitude. Bernheim published his famous book *De La Suggestion* (About Suggestion) in 1886, and in it he gave numerous instances of cures effected under hypnosis. The combined efforts of Bernheim and Liébault, following as they did upon the mark made by James Braid, effectively laid the foundations upon which modern hypnotherapy developed.

But, so far, nothing was known about the defensive value of symptoms or of the fact that they can often aid an individual to adjust to his difficulties. Hypnosis was simply used as a tool for crushing the patient's complaints and for this reason there were probably many more failures than there should have been. In 1880 Doctor Joseph Breuer, a Viennese GP, accidentally discovered that when one of his patients was persuaded to speak freely during a hypnotic trance, she underwent a deep emotional reaction and this was followed by the alleviation of many of her symptoms. Sigmund Freud later joined Breuer in conducting a full investigation of these results. The significance of this, was the subsequent change in the emphasis of hypnotherapy, from the mere removal of symptoms to the identification and eradication of their apparent causes. Later, unfortunately, Freud became disenchanted with hypnosis when he discovered that he was unable to induce very deep trance states, and he rejected it in favour of his own discovery of psychoanalysis.

This fact, together with the failure of hypnosis to produce a permanent cure for hysteria, nearly dealt the developing art a death blow; but the serious shortage of psychiatrists during the 1914-1918 war made a far briefer form of psychotherapy essential. Hypnotherapy was again revived and restored to popularity, and used effectively both in the direct removal of symptoms and in the reactivation of repressed traumatic experiences. War neuroses do in fact illustrate how very successful hypnotherapy can be, in the banishing of symptoms by means of reliving a shocking or horrifying experience. And the large scale of successes achieved in this way during and after the First World War, rightly regained the support for hypnotherapeutic suggestion which has continued to expand ever since.

Since the time mentioned, hypnotherapy has slowly gained ground and continues to establish an image of usefulness and acceptability. In 1952, the Hypnotism Act was passed, strictly defining the conditions under which hypnosis may be used in public demonstrations — thus effectively reducing the stage demonstrations of the art to a minimum. In addition, the Subcommittee of the British Medical Association's Psychological Group Committee, appointed in 1953 to look into the use of hypnotism in contemporary medicine, found much in favour of hypnosis as an adjunct to medicine. Findings under hypnosis had illustrated a great deal hitherto unknown about the working and the nature of the subconscious mind and its relationship to human behaviour. The Committee, although it warned against exaggerated claims being made on behalf of hypnotism, found it to be both useful and often the method of choice in treating a number of psychosomatic and psychoneurotic illnesses.

The Committee also found that hypnotism had a valuable rôle to play in surgery, dentistry and obstetrics, as an anaesthetic and as an analgesic (pain reliever), but emphasized that it should not be regarded as an independent speciality completely replacing other therapeutic methods.

Finally, the Committee suggested that the subject of hypnosis should be included in the courses on psychiatry held in Medical Schools and teaching hospitals, and possibly in courses of anaesthetics and obstetrics as well. It was in favour of further research being carried out into a number of aspects of the subject and outlined the fields meriting special clinical and laboratory investigation.

This Report has done a great deal to carve a permanent niche for hypnosis in modern medicine, although some of its recommendations are still waiting to be implemented. All the same, invaluable research into innovative techniques and treatment methods has been carried out during the past few years, particularly in the U.S.A., and hypnosis is gradually shedding its aura of mysticism and mystery.

I should point out that, in addition to the part hypnotherapy plays in modern medicine, its other major role consists of helping ordinary men and women to achieve a particular personal goal or to attain a greater degree of a socially desirable quality such as self-confidence. By 'ordinary' I mean people who are mentally and emotionally healthy but have a straightforward problem such as inability to lose weight, difficulty in ceasing to smoke, or an annoying habit such as blushing, stammering or excessive perspiration.

Strictly speaking, these personal problems are not 'medical' in nature, and while doctors may be involved in the suppression of symptoms (such as excessive nervous perspiration), or the provision of advice about an unhealthy condition (such as obesity) — the actual task of sticking to a prescribed diet or learning to overcome stress, resides strictly with the patient.

A hospital consultant or GP can advise a plump patient to avoid nibbling between meals, or prescribe beta-blocker drug therapy for sweating, palpitations, or a dry mouth. But all the advice in the world about the dangers of being overweight, can fall on deaf ears when the patient is excessively fond of chocolate. And not even the most hide-bound doctor would claim that the suppression of nervous symptoms was — in any circumstance — as desirable a measure as aiding the patient to overcome his causative personal difficulties.

This is the realm in which hypnotherapy comes into its own. For cigarette smoking, compensatory bingeing and fear of meeting people *can* be overcome with the help of a skilled therapist. And if the treatment is carried out successfully, the end-result will be far superior to the masking, or temporary abolition, of symptoms. The patient will have been helped to a deeper understanding of himself, his unwanted habit will have disappeared for good, and his self-confidence will have been given a justifiable boost by virtue of his having attained a personal goal.

There is, of course, a fine dividing line between a basically healthy individual who requires suggestions under hypnosis to reinforce his will-power, and one who is suffering from a slight but definable psychological problem such as occasional anxiety attacks or mild hypochondriasis. Where, for example, does a troublesome lack of self-confidence in the 'normal' person end, and a pathological fear of meeting people begin? And who is to say whether the man who appears obsessionally tidy — is neurotically so, or simply a variation on the theme of normality? Many skilled professionals, besides hypnotherapists, have to confront this problem. And to learn to solve it — if not in an absolute sense, philosophically speaking, at least in each instance where their balance of judgement will determine the diagnosis and treatment of a particular patient. Just as it is vital that a psychiatrist be able to identify the early signs of an illness such as schizophrenia, say, in a disturbed but dynamic and clearly intelligent young patient, in order to institute treatment — so, too, must a hypnotherapist be equipped to decide whether a troubled person is basically well; sick, but likely to benefit from hypnotherapy; or sick, and completely outside his field of practice.

This is where sound training, skill, judgement and an ethical code are called for. For just as orthodox medicine can cause a great deal of damage by misdiagnosing and thereby mistreating, so too, of course, can the practice of any other therapy. We will be looking in later chapters at the use of hypnotherapy in the treatment of psychological illness; and also at its use in helping people to achieve a particular objective.

1. What *is* Hypnosis?

This book is about the power hypnosis possesses to heal many forms of illness, both physical and mental. But in order to understand the nature of this power, it is essential that we are quite clear about what hypnosis is — as well as what it is not — and also how it works. It is not as a rule a very reliable practice to explain or define one phenomenon purely in terms of another, especially when neither concept is a familiar part of our everyday affairs or conversation, for it is possible to end up with one or several perfectly true statements, each as abstruse as the other, which do nothing whatsoever to clarify the situation!

Suggestibility
An idea, however, that is inseparable from that of hypnosis, is that of suggestion and suggestibility, so a good way to start is by explaining exactly what these are. Suggestion is a procedure by which a person willingly and totally accepts an idea or series of ideas propounded to him by another person, without subjecting it or them in the first place to examination by his critical faculties. As a corollary, suggestibility is the extent to which a person is able to make such an uncritical acceptance.

To be highly suggestible is to possess the type of mind which may — if you wish it to — respond to hypnosis very well. To be suggestible, is not at all the same thing as being either stupid or weak willed, as some people believe. It is, in fact, more difficult to hypnotize an unintelligent person than it is to hypnotize a mentally alert, intelligent one, as it is usually the latter individual who will be the more suggestible of the two.

The society in which we live, bombards us continually with all types of suggestion. And if this is news to you, because you have never really considered the matter critically before — this in itself is simply further evidence of the subtlety with which the suggestions are made to us. Your daily newspaper, whichever one you choose, has leading articles which are bound to reflect the opinion of the person writing them, and which seek to influence your opinion politically and/or socially by suggesting a particular viewpoint. A window-shopping spree, while it may extract no money from your purse at the time, is likely to reap some benefit to the retailers at a later date, when it 'suddenly occurs to you' that this carpet, that wallpaper, or the other curtain material, would look superb in your bedroom/lounge/kitchen.

Advertisements in magazines and on street hoardings, and even more so on television and radio, are powerful forms of suggestion which you may *think* you dismiss, because you don't really notice them and are not particularly interested in their messages anyway. Certainly when you are exposed to them, your mind may be very much engaged elsewhere, and this is specially true of radio 'jingle' advertisements which you maybe only hear while you are contending with busy traffic. At the end of your journey you may be quite unable to give an account of the products and companies which have jingled, sung, spoken and whistled their messages to you so intensively, for you have paid them no conscious attention.

But, in fact, commercial radio stations are an excellent way of feeding suggestions into the minds of audiences and they produce very real results for those who invest in advertising through them. This is because — and this is a very important point — the power of suggestion is enormously enhanced when it is directed at the subconscious rather than at the conscious mind.

Understanding basically what suggestion and suggestibility mean, we can now get on with defining hypnosis. Hypnosis is a state of consciousness in which suggestions are more readily accepted than they would be in a waking state, and lead to resultant action far more easily than they would if made to the alert, fully conscious person.

The purpose of the hypnotic state, from the hypnotist's point of view, is to increase the suggestibility of his subject. This always occurs when true hypnosis is induced, and the reason for it is that in an hypnotic state, the critical faculties are completely or partially suspended.

Hypnotic Trance

How does this happen? It happens because, when a person is in a hypnotic trance, his or her conscious mind — which is the seat of the critical faculties — is at rest, for the skill of the hypnotist lies in distracting the conscious mind of his subject so that he may deal directly with the suggestible subconscious. Just in case you think that the conscious mind is by far the more important of the two, and that its subconscious counterpart is a vague, shallow, primitive sort of region productive of dreams at night but not really playing any other part in our lives — you will be surprised to know that, on the contrary, the subconscious mind is by far the greater part.

Although normally we are unaware of its existence, the 'subconscious' is an immense storehouse of every one of our past experiences, thoughts, feelings and impressions, whether these are consciously remembered or long ago forgotten. And, in fact, of all the knowledge we have ever gleaned. A diagram (see figure 1) that accurately represents the relationship between the conscious mind and the subconscious, is that of an iceberg. The small tip, apparent to anyone in the vicinity, projecting from the surface of the water, is the conscious region. The vast, hidden, incalculable area below the surface — in a real iceberg constituting about nine tenths of it — on the psychological scale represents the subconscious territory.

Once the hypnotist has induced a state of hypnotic trance in his subject (and we will see how he does this in subsequent chapters) — what then? Does free access to his subject's undefended subconscious, give the unethical hypnotist an open sesame to run the full gamut of his harmful fantasies, and instil suggestions of unimaginable absurdity and chaos into the mind of his vulnerable subject? It is possible that a skilled and ill-intentioned hypnotist could cause severe harm to a highly suggestible person in whom he had induced a state of deep hypnosis. But I am not concerned here with immoral practitioners of an art which, like medicine, can only fairly be judged by the intentions, skill and achievements of the vast majority of those who practise it. Unethical hypnotherapists, like unethical physicians and surgeons, must exist, although I am pleased to say that I have never personally encounted one.

So let me say, here and now, that I am discussing hypnotherapy in the light of my own experience of hypnotherapists practising

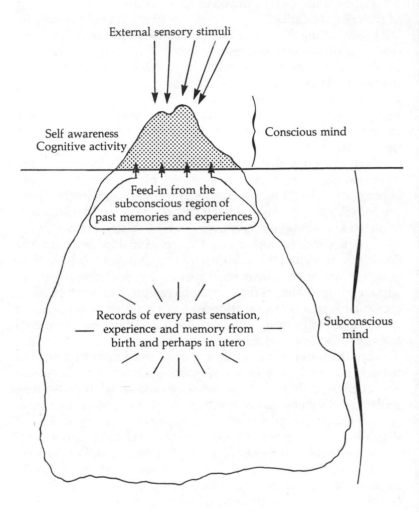

Figure 1: The Mental Iceberg

in this country, and of my own personal colleagues in the medical profession. And the aim of the hypnotherapist is to discover the cause of his patient's problems and to eradicate them wherever possible.

The Power of Hypnotism

A number of serious misconceptions exist about the practice of hypnosis as a form of therapy, however, and it is one of the aims of this book to dispel them. Firstly, in contradistinction to one popular belief, no hypnotherapist can 'make' his subject or patient behave in a manner that is foreign to his (or her) basic nature. We hear many stories of stage hypnotists inviting members of their audience to participate in staged trance induction, and suggesting to them while in a hypnotic trance that they are, for example, domestic or farm animals — with the result that the subjects hop, spring and crawl around the stage to the amusement of the rest of the audience, barking, yelping, miaowing and braying like so many dogs, cats and donkeys.

Indeed such feats have been performed. It was a less common feat to see performed years ago than many people now suppose, and fortunately it is not seen often nowadays. What the stage hypnotist was *not* doing, though, was causing his subjects to behave in a manner that was foreign to their inmost wishes or beliefs. You may dispute this, on the grounds that it is not within human nature to wish to make a fool of oneself, by pretending to be a domestic animal just to provide a laugh for an unsympathetic crowd. But there must be that within the personal make-up of the subject, that sufficiently concurs with the wishes of the hypnotist, to enable the hypnotic suggestions to take effect. In other words — people on whom such suggestions work, possess a basic desire to act the fool in front of a public audience. If they did not want to behave in an extroverted fashion before a large number of people, no hypnotist on earth, however skilled, could make them do so.

It is quite impossible for a hypnotist, however cunning, to urge his subject to a form of conduct or behaviour unnatural to him, either while in a state of hypnotic trance or afterwards by means of post-hypnotic suggestion. So, do remember from the start that the subject remains in charge. The hypnotherapist can suggest and guide; but he cannot order or force.

The Need for Rapport

One factor that is helpful to the successful induction of the hypnotic state, and essential to its curative application, is a state of rapport between subject and hypnotherapist. Given that the subject is reasonably intelligent, alert and co-operative, and the hypnotist experienced, competent and sufficiently au fait with his subject's personality to avoid making unacceptable hypnotic suggestions to him — a feeling of empathy between subject and hypnotist is still essential for a hypnotic trance of lasting value to be induced.

Even given a good degree of empathy between the two, it is still the patient rather than the hypnotherapist who does the bulk of the work! He does this by the use of his subconscious mind, which, as we have noted, does not possess any kind of critical faculty. We may be tempted to say that any work the patient does, is very passive in nature but it is the subconscious mind of the patient not of his therapist, which receives and subsequently acts upon the constructive suggestions made to it.

As we have seen, the subconscious is a store house of memories, good and bad, and while not possessing the ability to appraise a situation it is programmed by past experiences to accept that which is 'good' for it, and reject that which is 'bad'. So a suggestion that a subject is going to behave in a way that is very much to his own detriment and which does nothing to satisfy a basic urge (such as that of 'showing off', in the case of the stage subjects), will be rejected — and the trance state very likely broken into the bargain. The subject remains in control throughout the entire operation — and at no point does he surrender his will power to the dominant power of the hypnotist.

Other factors influencing a subject's susceptibility besides a basic level of intelligence and willingness to co-operate, to the induction of a trance, are his age, sex, personality type and the presence or absence of mental illness. *Sex* — although many hypnotists find no obvious difference in suggestibility between the two sexes, a number claim that women are the easier to hypnotize. One trial conducted to investigate the matter, though, came to the conclusion that 'women college students with a positive attitude towards hypnosis' were better hypnotic subjects than their male counterparts. But no real reason for this finding was discovered. [1]

Personality type — a lot of interest has been shown in this factor by workers researching hypnosis. It is difficult to make a hard and fast rule about it, but many people agree that the model personality type is the one described by Gill and Brenman. They postulated it to be: 'one possessing an intense subconscious need for passivity, at the same time being aggressively demanding'. This hypothetical 'ideal hypnotic subject' would also have a tendency to 'oral conflicts' (which I will explain all about later), and these would more than likely express themselves as 'eating illnesses', either bingeing or starving to a point of anorexia.

Other workers investigating personality types and suggestibility to hypnosis, have found that the average non-athletic individual is *more* likely to make a good hypnotic subject than the man or woman who plays a great deal of sport or who is very athletically gifted.

Again the extent to which a person temperamentally resembles his or her parent of the *opposite* sex, is known to be linked with suggestibility. The greater the resemblance, the greater the degree of suggestibility; but if the subject resembles in temperament his or her parent of the *same* sex, then they will be a good hypnotic subject only if the parent is! Someone who resembles neither parent, with respect to matters such as recreational pursuits, type of work or employment etc., is likely to be difficult to hypnotize.

These research findings are interesting, which is why I thought they were worth mentioning here. But in practice it makes very little difference, when you go along to see a hypnotherapist, which — if either — parent you personally resemble. The therapist will be much more concerned with taking a full history of the problems currently bothering you, to worry himself about whether you are similar to your father, or dissimilar to your mother, except in so far as these factors may have a bearing on your present problems.

Mental Illness
We will go into the nature of 'the neuroses' (i.e, neurotic illness) in a later chapter — examples are anxiety, and mild to moderate depression. A person suffering from one of these illnesses is neither more nor less likely, on the strength of his complaint, to make a good hypnotic subject. People with chronic psychotic illnesses (again, see later), seem almost impervious to attempts to hypnotize them.[2] Individuals suffering from an acute form of psychosis, however, can either be very good hypnotic subjects, or extremely poor.

Age — this makes a difference to suggestibility. In 1887, Liébault showed children between the ages of seven and fourteen years to be the most susceptible age group. Many people who have studied the subject, feel that degree of suggestibility is more related to the person's ability to rôle play, i.e, enter in his imagination into a situation that the therapist creates, than to actual age in years. As a general rule of thumb, though, children make better hypnotic subjects than do older people.

It can be noted here that nationality does not seem to affect suggestibility one way or the other. The average hypnotherapist can expect to find that between eighty and ninety per cent of the patients he sees are hypnotizable to a useful level. Somewhere between thirteen and twenty-six per cent of the population as a whole, are capable of entering into a very deep hypnotic trance, whereas around sixty-six per cent of them, are capable of light trance induction.

Dissimilarity to Brainwashing
Another misconception about hypnosis, is that suggesting ideas to a person's subconscious mind in the course of a hypnotic trance, is similar to the process of brainwashing. There is no similarity whatever, in theory or in practice, between the processes of brainwashing and using hypnosis as a form of therapy. Brainwashing is carried out upon victims, not upon patients; and the intentions of those performing the brainwashing are cruel, intent only upon achieving their own ends, and unaffected by the degree of mental and physical suffering involved in bringing about the change they wish to take place in their victims' minds.

Conscious resistance is broken down, in the process of brainwashing, by prolonged exposure to systematic indoctrination or mental pressure aimed at causing an alteration in the victim's behaviour pattern or opinion. New ideas are implanted by force and in opposition to the subject's, or victim's, will. There is no question of the establishment of a genuine, sincere rapport, or of co-operation between oppressor and victim, or — of course — of working to benefit the latter.

Hypnotherapy is conducted with the acquiescence and co-operation of the subject or patient. Generally an altered mode of behaviour, either long or short term, follows upon successful hypnotic suggestion, and upon successful brainwashing. Here, the similarity begins and ends.

Dissimilarity to Sleeping State

Another misconception about the hypnotic trance, is that it is very similar to the sleeping state. New subjects, or patients, experiencing hypnosis for the first time, frequently believe that something highly dramatic is going to happen and that they will lose consciousness altogether in such a manner that when they finally 'come to' — they will remember very little, if anything, of what has occurred. Consequently, when they experience real life trance induction for the first time — and note to their consternation that they remain fully aware of all stages of the procedure from start to finish, they often complain that they have not been hypnotized at all and maybe even cancel further therapy appointments in the mistaken belief that they are 'incapable of being hypnotized'.

As we have just seen, between eight and nine people out of every ten in this part of the world, are capable of experiencing a sufficiently deep trance for them to benefit from hypnotherapeutic treatment, so the person who really does remain immune to trance induction at the hands of a skilled therapist, is the 'odd man out'. The trouble lies, not in the failure of trance to occur, but in misconceived ideas on the behalf of the subject, preventing treatment from progressing any further.

There is little true similarity between the sleeping state, and a state of hypnotic trance. When you fall asleep, you are oblivious of all that is around you — and if someone came into your room and talked to you in a sufficiently quiet tone for you to remain asleep, you obviously would not know, or remember, a word that had been spoken. You would in no sense be in charge of the situation, and certainly not in any sense able to exert any type of control. You may or may not remember details of the event after it had occurred — this definitely would not happen if your state of true sleep had remained undisturbed.

When you go into a state of trance you are aware of everything that is going on around you. We will see exactly what happens, and what it feels like, in the next chapter, but suffice it to say here that the most notable feeling during the procedure is one of remoteness. You feel vague and detached, and your eyelids feel heavy and inclined to close. But you do not go 'right off' as you do during a five minute doze after Sunday lunch, and you are capable afterwards of giving a precise account of all that has happened and all that has been said to you.

Hypnotism may be rather less dramatic than films, TV shows and novels lead you to believe — but it is capable of having far reaching effects that can greatly benefit the patient who is co-operative and receptive in the hands of an experienced and skilled hypnotherapist. So let us take a look in the following chapter at how these beneficial effects can be achieved.

2. What Actually Happens

Since we are concerned with the use of hypnosis as a form of treatment in this book, as opposed to the performance of hypnotic stage techniques for the purposes of public entertainment, from this point onwards I shall refer to hypnotherapists and patients rather than hypnotists and subjects. The methods and techniques are basically the same, of course, whatever the purpose to which trance induction is being put — but it stands to reason that each of the two types of practitioner approaches his job in a rather different manner from the other.

Let us suppose that *you* are considering a visit to a hypnotherapist, and let us further suppose that your problem is a straightforward one. You have no serious psychological neurosis requiring analysis and no deeply injurious emotional traumas in your past history — what you really need, is some straightforward, effective help in losing weight. Obesity and overeating are extremely common problems, and although there is often a serious underlying cause for such eating diseases as anorexia nervosa and bulimia, simply eating too much because you love food and cannot resist it does not imply some serious, forgotten psychological problem in earlier life.

You will either have been recommended to your therapist by your GP or a friend, or have looked up the name of one living in your neighbourhood in Yellow Pages. The usual length of a session is one hour — and the fees range from £7.50 per visit to as much as £15 or £20. Do not ask, when you telephone for an appointment, how many sessions you are going to need. No hypnotherapist can tell you that, although he may well form an idea of the length of treatment required once he as met you and discussed your problem with you, and placed you under hypnotic trance for the first time.

The First Session

The usual duration of each visit is about one hour, but it is normal for the first session to take a little longer, for the therapist will wish to take down some personal details, and the story of your current problem, and ascertain whether there are likely to be attendant psychological problems below the surface. He will also want to make sure — for your sake and his — that you do not fall into the limited category of people whom it is very unwise to subject to hypnosis. And he will wish to discover how strongly motivated you are to overcome your problem, whether you have been hypnotized before, and whether you entertain any secret fears, doubts or misconceptions about hypnotherapy and what it involves. For fear or resentment provide a very real barrier to the success of hypnotic treatment.

So for the sake of simplicity, we are supposing that your biggest problem in life is the fact that you are two and half stone overweight, due to an excessively sweet tooth and the inability to say 'no' to bars of chocolate and cream doughnuts. The hypnotherapist will first of all ask your age, full name and address, and the type of work you do; and then include questions aimed specifically at your problem such as the times of day when your resistance is lowest, the availability of tempting snacks etc. He may give some practical advice on how to avoid particularly difficult situations, and then proceed to find out the other information I have outlined above.

All the time your hypnotherapist is asking you questions, he will be trying to achieve several aims simultaneously. He will genuinely wish to put you at your ease, for, as we have seen, a good rapport is essential to successful hypnotherapy. He will be attempting to obtain the other information I have mentioned as this is essential to the practice of the art. Thirdly, he will be assessing the possibility of any risk — to you or to himself — in his proceeding with hypnosis. A properly trained hypnotherapist will have had a sound training in psychology and while hypnotherapy is extremely useful in dealing with many psychological problems it has carefully definable limitations and boundaries.

Unsuitable Subjects

Certain degrees of pronounced hysteria are best left to a psychiatrist, as are a number of the psychotic illnesses such as schizophrenia. Few hypnotherapists take on patients suffering from grand mal epilepsy, or people diagnosed as insane. You may also be surprised to learn that the risks involved in hypnotizing a member of the public are a two way affair. A number of people — more often women than men — possessing an unstable temperament and a tendency to hysteria, are in a position to make life troublesome and dangerous for their hypnotherapist. A hysterical patient whose hypnotic trance recollections get mixed up in her mind with wish fulfilment, can make all manner of accusations against her therapist if it should come into her mind to do so. This is one of the reasons why male hypnotherapists (and doctors and other types of therapist) employ female receptionist staff who act as chaperones whenever necessary — and why some male hypnotherapists record the entire consultation whenever they interview and treat a female patient solo.

Do not underestimate this point, though. The hypnotherapist, especially the man who practises alone, and is not always equipped with a lady receptionist or nurse, is in far more potential danger from his patients than they could ever be from him!

Suggestibility Tests
When the hypnotherapist has talked to you for a bit, he may well wish to carry out one or two suggestibility tests, so that he can ascertain whether you are likely to be an easy or a difficult hypnotic subject. In one such test, you will be asked to hold your right arm, for example, out straight in front of you and the therapist will take its weight by placing his hands at your forearm and elbow, asking you as he does so, to relax the muscles of your arm completely. He will tell you to indicate when you are sure that your muscles are relaxed and, without warning you, will withdraw his supporting grip.

If you have achieved relaxation, then your arm will fall heavily to your side. If your relaxation has been incomplete, your arm will descend slowly to your side. And if you have remained tense, then your arm will remain where it is, suspended in the air.

The swaying test, is another test which reveals how suggestible you are. You will be asked to stand upright with your feet together and your eyes closed. Your therapist will stand behind you, and place his fingers on the back of your neck, explaining what he is doing and then telling you that as he draws his fingers back, away from you and towards himself, you will sway backwards with the motion of his hands. He will assure you that there is no danger of your falling for, the moment you start to do so, he will catch you. If his suggestion has been given in an authoritative and convincing way, you will very likely do exactly as he has foretold.

A third test of your likely susceptibility to hypnotic suggestion, is a sitting-down one. You will be asked to settle back comfortably in your armchair, relax your arms and stretch your legs out in front of you, so that they rest easily and naturally on the floor. As soon as you are relaxed, you will be told to keep your arms and legs still, and that when you close your eyes you will be unable to leave your chair and get up. If you are reasonably suggestible and relaxed, and assuming your hypnotherapist is a skilled one, you will find yourself unable to move.

Trance Induction

Having performed suggestibility tests, the hypnotherapist is then in a position to start inducing a state of hypnosis. The curtains will be drawn and the room will be comfortably warm. You will be asked to make yourself as comfortable as possible — and if you have neglected to do so, do ask to visit the bathroom at this point if you find you need to do so. Don't be shy, for the therapist wishes to achieve results as much as you wish it, and it is very difficult indeed to be receptive to hypnotic suggestion when your bladder is bursting!

Then settle back in your armchair as directed, or make yourself comfortable on the couch, and listen to what the therapist says to you. Give him all your attention and try to prevent other thoughts from entering your mind. Don't try too hard, though, for this in itself can be an obstacle. Just relax all your muscles and concentrate thoroughly without in any sense straining. He will start to talk to you in an unobtrusive but authoritative manner, and you will find that his words flow smoothly and easily without awkward interruptions and constrained pauses.

These are some of the techniques he may employ to induce a light state of hypnosis. Fixing his attention, and yours, on the various parts of your body and working systematically upwards from your feet (first one, then the other) — to the top of your head (by way of every part of you, including neck muscles, throat, facial muscles, tongue and forehead) — your therapist may suggest that the muscles in the regions mentioned are feeling warm, comfortable and relaxed, and that they are getting heavy. He will suggest that you feel tired, relaxed and unwilling to move any part of yourself. Talking about your left forearm, for example, he will say something along these lines: 'The muscles of your left forearm are getting tired and heavy. They are warm, and comfortably relaxed, and you start to notice a faint pleasant tingling sensation in them as a feeling of warmth, comfort and relaxation creeps slowly up them from your wrist to your elbow; and this sensation of warmth, comfort and relaxation starts to affect your left upper arm . . .'

The therapist will repeat certain suggestive words time and again, and use a quiet and monotonous tone of voice. Having directed your attention to every part of your body, he will then suggest that you are warm, peaceful, comfortable, weary and utterly relaxed and that it would be far too much trouble for you to do anything at all, but to continue to listen to his voice. If the induction has been successful you will find that all your muscles, including the 'difficult' ones such as those of your eyelids, lips and tongue, will be gently relaxed, just as they are when you are in bed and on the verge of sleep, and neither tense nor twitching uncontrollably. Your eyes will be closed and you will be feeling comfortable, relaxed and dreamy.

Another method your hypnotherapist may use to induce the trance state, is to tell you to close your eyes and 'look upwards' with your eyes closed at a point on your forehead where he has placed his forefinger. You cannot of course 'see' this point, or anything else; but by attempting to keep your fixed 'gaze' on the area of skin he is touching, you will be having to concentrate very hard which is of great assistance to the induction. Meanwhile, your therapist will instruct you to count backwards quietly to yourself, say from three hundred to one — and while you are thus doubly occupied, will suggest that 'with every breath that you breathe in, you are inhaling a pleasant smelling gas that is sending you to sleep', and that 'with every breath you exhale, you are breathing out worries, stress and tension'.

A very large number of effective induction techniques exist. A third that your therapist may favour, will involve your settling down comfortably in your chair or on the couch, and staring at the tip of a pencil, light or small object held some eight inches in front of your eyes. You will be asked to stare unwaveringly

at the object — and if your eyes happen to wander from the point
your therapist will immediately draw your attention to the fact.
While you are staring fixedly at the object, the therapist will make
verbal suggestions to you along the following lines:

'Take a deep breath and blow it out of your lungs, slowly and
gently. Continue to breathe quietly and comfortably. Let your
body go limp, and relax totally and completely all over in every
muscle. You will start to feel that your eyes are becoming very,
very tired. And that your eyelids are feeling heavier and heavier.
You will want to blink . . . you feel warm and relaxed, contented
and tired . . . your eyelids are becoming very, very heavy . . .
they are wanting to close . . . and as soon as they close, you will
fall into a deep, deep sleep.'

As you inevitably close your eyes, the therapist may then bid
you 'go to sleep' and your eyes will from that point onwards
remain closed. By this time you will be in a light hypnotic state.

The Trance State

What exactly has happened to bring this state of trance about?
Because your attention has been fixed on different parts of your
body, a small object, or a spot you cannot see on your forehead
etc., you have relaxed into the state known as hypnosis and the
therapist's voice alone is carried by certain nerve fibres in the
brain which normally carry sound, thoughts and messages. Since
the therapist's voice is the only stimulus which is receiving
attention, the suggestions he makes are in a position to overcome
all feelings of anxiety, fear, anger and other emotion. The voice
of your therapist, in other words, has become 'locked' to your
mind at the level of the subconscious realm. And this, as we have
seen, is where all your past experiences and feelings are stored.

Is your therapist bound to know whether you have entered
a hypnotic trance or not? If you have, then you will look extremely
relaxed at this stage, and your breathing will be slow and regular,
and you will remain perfectly still unless and until he asks you
to open your eyes. Your own feeling is one of deep and pleasant
relaxation, and a strong disinclination to make any sort of effort,
for your body and limbs are tired and heavy and there may be
sensations of numbness, tingling or dullness in your arms or
hands. Some people feel a floating or light sensation, and very
commonly an impression of detachment and distance from their
surrounding environment.

At this stage, before making the chosen suggestions to you designed to help you with your particular problem, your hypnotherapist may wish to deepen your trance. There are many different ways of achieving this, and they are basically extensions of the induction technique. One method is to tell you that your hand, which is lying quiescent on the couch or chair arm, is growing lighter and lighter, and that it will eventually rise in the air without your conscious effort and touch your face — at which point your trance will be considerably deepened.

This device is very useful, since the therapist can utilize it both to ascertain that you are actually in an hypnotic trance and simultaneously employ it to deepen the state of that trance.

The Scope of the Deep Trance State

Having achieved the desired degree of trance — or having induced as deep a degree as the patient is capable of sustaining — the therapist can do a number of things. At a very deep level of trance he can, for example, induce anaesthesia to enable a surgical operation to be performed, a tooth to be extracted, or a labour and delivery to progress to a successful conclusion without pain being experienced by the mother. If your therapist decides you are capable of this degree of trance, he will probably effect what is known as 'glove anaesthesia' in one or other of your hands. Pricks of the skin covering that hand by a sharp pin or needle, will fail to produce the usual withdrawal response, since you will be aware of no pain or discomfort whatever.

It is also possible after sufficient trance depth has been induced to affect the function of the patient's various muscle groups, organs and glands by means of carefully directed and powerful suggestions, and to implant ideas that will help to overcome the practice of a habit which the patient wishes to be rid of, such as smoking, stammering, blushing, nailbiting or overeating. A usual way of achieving this end is by means of *post-hypnotic suggestion*. If for instance your therapist does this for you, in order to dissuade you from bingeing on chocolates and cream cakes, he may say something like:

'From this time onwards, you will not be tempted to eat chocolates or cream cakes. You may see them and want them — but if you pick one up and put it in your mouth, you will get the disgusting taste of sewage on doing so. It will taste, smell and feel so revolting to you, that you will not be tempted to repeat the experience. But if you should forget what it was like and place one of these substances in your mouth again, exactly the same experience will be repeated. You will be sickened by the taste, smell and feel of stinking, oozing, slimy sewage in your mouth and on your tongue and you will spit out the offending object and never wish to repeat the horrible experience again.'

You may think this suggestion is worded rather strongly. But if overeating happens really to be one of your problems you will know that it is a very hard habit to break and that you do in fact need all the concentrated help you can get, truly to wean you from over-indulging in this way.

Sometimes, more than the removal of superficial symptoms and annoying habit patterns is required, and the preliminary case history points to the presence of an underlying neurotic illness. Hypnotherapy goes well beyond the suppression of smoking, biting one's nails or having tummy upsets prior to interviews or examinations, and probes the subconscious mind of the patient for the key to the problem by bringing to the surface, i.e, to the conscious mind of the subject, forgotten memories or the emotional reliving of past traumatic events.

If carefully carried out by a skilled hypnotherapist, it can solve the problem of the patient's illness and thereby rid him or her of troublesome behaviour patterns that caused him to seek hypnotherapy in the first place. In order to understand how this comes about, we have to take a look at what the human mind is, how it works, and how psychological abnormalities come about.

3. The Mind and How It Works

We saw earlier the similarity between the structure of the mind and that of an iceberg — at least with respect to pictorial representation! The superficial and visible tip of the latter is equivalent to the conscious mind, and is involved with our every day thoughts, decisions, and activities. The submerged nine-tenths of the berg are equivalent to our subconscious mind, and access can be gained to this region through the medium of hypnosis.

The Conscious Mind

We owe this concept of mental structure to Freud. To him, consciousness (i.e, our every day awareness) represented a small part only of the complete picture of psychic anatomy, and accounted for a correspondingly small part of total mental activity. Just as the images one sees in a mirror, are sharply defined, fleeting and readily apparent, so the contents of our conscious minds can be likened to reflections seen in the full light of day in a highly mirrored surface. For the conscious mind reflects the constantly varying pattern of every thought, feeling, reaction and desire of which we are aware, at any particular moment in time.

And just as the images you can view in a mirror are limited by the shape and size of the reflecting surface, so the extent of our conscious thoughts is bounded by our ability to cope with or contain several different thoughts, ideas and feelings simultaneously. The chief feature of our conscious mind is the propensity of awareness, and the data with which it deals emanate from two origins. One of these is all the sensory stimuli which bombard us continually during our waking hours from our surrounding environment — that is, the sum total of all the sights, sounds, smells, sensations and tastes that we encounter. And the other is the association our conscious mind makes between the sensory stimuli we are receiving and recollections of comparable past events.

You may, for instance, be fully consciously preoccupied with writing a letter to a friend. As you write, you are aware of what you wish to say, of the contents of her last letter or conversation with you, and at the same time of your feelings towards her as someone productive of a certain degree of emotion. The name of your friend reminds you of your letter, your news, and the fact that you wish to write. The sight of her letter on the table in front of you, will have the same effect. And any predominant emotion associated in your conscious mind with her, will be claiming a portion of your awareness too.

At the same time, the sensation of a finely turned, new wooden pen in your hand, will evoke a memory very close to consciousness, of the trip out last Saturday week which you took to a nearby town where you bought your pen — and of the attendant pleasure you derived from the company you kept that day — say with your husband or wife, or maybe you were alone and enjoyed yourself for that very reason.

While your consciousness is busy dealing with these stimuli, a delivery van calls at the door and interrupts your flow of thought — or, pleasanter to contemplate, a delicious aroma of roast chicken and herb stuffing assails you and immediately your conscious mind associates the stimulus with the memory of when you last ate — and you realize that you are extremely hungry!

Alternatively your sense of smell may detect that leeks are being cooked downstairs. You cannot bear them, and immediately remember unhappy days at boarding school when you faced cold leeks for an entire afternoon in an effort to eat the wretched things. The direction of your conscious thoughts will be rerouted through a few minutes of childhood recollections.

A third way of regarding the conscious mind, in addition to comparing it with the tip of an iceberg or a highly polished mirror, is to see it as a screen on to which the moving images of a film are being projected. The reel on which the film has been made may be lengthy and involved, and contain many interesting pieces of information, emotive scenes etc; but the only part of it that we can be aware of, at any one moment in time, is that portion passing in front of the lens, and being projected and focussed upon the screen.

The Subconscious Mind

Our subconscious mind is the reel, for it contains a record of every past scene and contact with which we have been involved. But in order for us to gain access to this fascinating record, it must be projected on to the screen of our conscious awareness. And because that screen is limited in size and shape, so only a very limited portion of the reel can be viewed (i.e., experienced) at any one moment.

To the conscious and subconscious (or unconscious) mental regions, has been added a third one termed 'preconsciousness'. This is the store house of easily accessible memories, as opposed to the subconscious mind 'proper', which contains forgotten or repressed thoughts, feelings and memories, together with the primitive and basic drives and instincts which strongly influence our actions whether we are aware of them or not.

Sigmund Freud

Much of Freud's work was involved with the conflicts that arise between the conscious mind and the 'unconscious instincts', suppressed memories, and so on. For he believed that mental illness resulted from such conflicts, or rather, from a failure to resolve them satisfactorily. Freud (1856-1939) was first of all a distinguished neurologist, and practised as such before directing his attention to mental function, thereby becoming a pioneer of both modern psychology and psychiatry. The art of psychoanalysis originated with him, and this form of treatment attempts to bring suppressed conflicts and fears to the consciousness of the patient, with beneficial results to many. Many hypnotherapists are mainly Freudian in their view of psychology and the development of mental illness, and their analytical treatment of neurotic illness ('hypno-analysis') owes a great deal to Freud's psychoanalytic theory.

Both Freud and the hypnotist Breuer (see page 18) were in agreement that finding a specific memory association which would account for a troublesome neurotic symptom, resulted in the ebbing of the painful emotions concerned. Many observations which Freud made about early forgotten painful memories pointed to a common factor in many of them — and this was the experience by the individual of some degree of sexual trauma in childhood. For sexual trauma we should not jump to the obvious conclusion that actual and overt 'sex trauma' was meant — i.e., the kind of thing appearing in the newspapers from time to time about the sexual molestation of a child by an adult. To Freud, sex was a very wide term indeed and his theories about it underlay a great deal of his observations about the developing psyche. It is really preferable to substitute the word 'sexuality', so that at least we form an impression of a whole aspect of maturation rather than the confined idea of the sexual act itself.

Most people to whom Freud is a familiar name, associate the terms 'ego', 'id' and 'super-ego' with him; his work *The Ego and the Id* appeared in 1922, and it presented a picture of personality development along the following lines:

A newborn baby requires nourishment, love and security in order to survive, and its instinctual drives are directed exclusively at obtaining and retaining these factors. It is dominated by the 'id' principle at this stage, for the primitive impulses act without any form of direction from a superior guiding principle.

As soon as the infant discovers that the realities and frustrations of his external environment are forces to be reckoned with, his self or 'ego' is formed from the primeval emotional mass and its chief function is to test out reality so that the infant's efforts and reactions can be more profitably directed — and therefore successful — in achieving satisfaction. Later when a growing awareness of the opinions and restrictions of society start to dawn, the 'super-ego' or conscience principle starts to come into being.

Carl Gustav Jung

Carl Gustav Jung (1875-1961) split off from the group of Freudian disciples to which he had been attached in 1913, chiefly because, like Adler, he disagreed with what he felt was Freud's undue emphasis upon sexuality. Words common to every day speech, such as 'introvert', 'extravert' and 'complex', originated with Jung, as did the theory of archetypes and the doctrine of psychological truth. There is no need to expand upon these principles of Jungian psychology here, but because of the significance attached to the subconscious mind by Freud and consequently by many hypnotherapists, Jung's idea of this realm of the human psyche is worth mentioning.

Besides the contents attributed by Freud to the subconscious (i.e., the primitive instincts, and forgotten memories, experiences and impressions) Jung thought it to contain aspects of mental life 'which have been neglected in the course of development';

unapprehended experiences and ideas, forgotten about because they have lost a 'certain energic value'; and finally the collective or racial unconscious as well. For the personal unconscious as Freud saw it, was according to Jung a relatively small part of the total mass of unconscious material. At a lower level that the personal unconscious, Jung placed the collective or racial unconscious, because it contained the sum total of myths and beliefs of the race to which the individual belonged. The deepest levels of the collective unconscious, Jung named the 'universal unconscious', shared by all human beings and even by his primate and animal ancestry.

Alfred Adler

Alfred Adler, another member of the post-Freudian school to develop his own system of psychology, is worth mentioning in passing. The basic principle underlying the Adlerian approach, can best be expressed in his own words:

'To be a human being means the possession of a feeling of inferiority that is constantly pressing on towards its own conquest.' Adler came to think as he did probably as a result of his interest in the body's ability to compensate for organic damage. For instance, an injured or diseased kidney or lung may be compensated for by an increase in functional capacity of its healthy counterpart organ. He regarded childhood as a time when all human beings experience strong inferiority and he thought that this was so, regardless of whether the child was loved, protected and wanted, or unloved, ill-treated and abused.

He felt that all children as they develop, work out their own particular strategy for coping with family relationships as seen from their own point of view, in order to compensate for their innate feelings of inadequacy and inferiority. It is upon this 'lifestyle' that the adult character is founded. The resultant nature of this character would depend upon the individual's physical constitution, his economic and social standing, his sex, his level of education, family interrelationships etc.

Adler saw three possible results of the individual's attempts to overcome the unpleasing inferiority impressions he entertained. The first was *successful compensation* which accounts for people who develop normally into happy and healthy, well-balanced men and women, able to deal without undue trouble with life's three greatest challenges as Adler saw them, namely work, sex and society. The second possible outcome was *overcompensation*, when the efforts are excessive and thereby become too apparent and lead to a certain amount of maladjustment, such as what we all know as the 'small man syndrome'.

The third possible outcome, was *the retreat into illness as a means of obtaining power*. One of the most significant things Adler wrote, was: 'Every neurosis can be understood as an attempt to free oneself from a feeling of inferiority in order to gain a feeling of superiority.' These words put one very much in mind of aspects of the hysterical personality and of the hypochondriac, as will be apparent when we come to look at these neurotic traits and how they come into being.

One sometime gets the impression when starting to read books on psychology — in particular, accounts of how it has developed — that just as 'all paths lead to Rome', according to a number of theologians — so most aspects of the subject are ultimately traceable to Sigmund Freud. The reason for this common observation is surely that, rather than merely discovering facts, Freud radically affected the way in which we regard human beings generally and ourselves in particular. His approach to human psychology changed it from a non-developing no-man's land subject related to philosophy and physics, to a dynamic and flourishing science in its own right, based firmly upon biological observation and extending without pretension into the realm of sociology. He explained behaviour in positive, goal-directed terms — and the tenets he postulated as forming the basis of his psychological system, are tried and tested and continue to work perfectly satisfactorily.

As I mentioned, hypnotherapists adhere in the main to Freudian psychology, but others do of course have a preference for Jung, Adler and other more recent schools of thought. At first glance, the different theories may seem to you to be severely at variance with one another, but it is a surprising fact that, in a group of therapists belonging to different psychological disciplines, there is usually agreement rather than dispute among them with respect to the personality type of a particular patient, the diagnosis of his problem(s), and the treatment suitable to him. And from the patient's point of view, it is of academic interest only whether his therapist is a confirmed Freudian, a follower of Adlerian techniques, or of established Jungian convictions. Provided of course that the therapist can help him to overcome his unwanted habit pattern, or diagnose and treat his neurotic illness.

To achieve results, there is no doubt that a hypnotherapist has to choose to study and to follow a particular psychological system and to stick to it. Freudian psychology suits hypnotherapists very well, since his observations and approach work reliably and provide a good framework in which to discuss mental function. Freud also gives a clear picture of a likely mode of early psychical development — both to normality and to a range of psychological aberrations which are commonly encountered by practising hypnotherapists. We will ultimately be looking at case histories of patients and examining their problems, to see how they can be treated and helped by hypnotherapy.

In the next chapter we take a look at early sexuality in the newborn baby and small child and discover how common problems arising later in life can result from mishandling during that period.

4. Oral Conflicts

Psychological problems arise in childhood. Most systems of psychology agree with one another about that, and to Freud they stemmed from the moment of birth. All human beings when they are tiny, experience conflicts of one sort or another, and in the majority of people these constitute just a healthy stimulus to normal growth and development — since whatever the odds, most of us do develop into reasonably balanced 'normal' people. Some infants, however, face conflicts so great that they do not succeed in resolving them satisfactorily, and the conflicts give rise to neurotic illnesses (the neuroses) later in life.

A number of factors determine our success or failure in overcoming the turmoils of early infancy. One of these is the type of personality we inherit from our parents. This plays an undeniably important role, for while our physical and emotional circumstances as babies are to a great extent responsible for our ultimate attainment (or failure to attain) harmony and balance, genetically inherited tendencies to, for example, an anxious or a depressive personality also help to determine the outcome of our personality development.

The relationships that exist between us and our parents, however, and between us and other family members, are critical in determining our future happiness, as are characteristics of the material environment around us. Physical deprivation of nourishment, for instance, will threaten a small baby's sense of security as surely as the negligent behaviour of an unloving mother.

The Basic Instincts
Freud identified two great driving forces or instincts — the drive towards *self-preservation* and the drive towards *procreation*. He

termed the latter *'sexual energy'* or *libido*, and thought that in many of us, this energy is bottled up or repressed in our subconscious minds, denied its proper expression by the censorial attitudes of society. Although when he initially used the word 'sex', Freud meant what you and I normally mean by it in everyday conversation, he soon started to use the term in a much broader sense to embrace all pleasurable physical sensations, as well as feelings such as affection, pleasure derived from a pursuit of, and the bonds of, friendship.

He felt justified in extending the definition of 'sex' or 'sexuality' so widely because he felt that it was a force or energy drive expressing itself in many different ways and manifesting itself in previously unsuspected channels. Homosexuality, for instance, is an example of sexual feeling directed at a member of one's own sex instead of at a member of the opposite sex, and in some people the sex drive is directed towards him or her own self, or towards animals, or even towards inanimate objects. Secondly, Freud noticed that the mouth and the anus could equally well serve as the object of sexual activity, besides the genital organs; and lastly he noticed a similarity between the behaviour of babies and that of adult perverts. For example, thumb sucking, delight in showing off the naked body or in looking at it as a means of obtaining sexual gratification, and fascination with the processes of urination and defaecation.

The Libido

Having postulated that emotional problems stem from early conflicts, Freud studied the libido in great detail because he thought that it was within the realm of repressed sexual instincts rather than within that of threatened self-preservation that the origins of the conflicts were likely to lie. Regarding the mouth, anus and genitals, which he noticed were the sources of a great deal of sexual satisfaction, Freud suggested that the development of sexuality passed through three definite chronological stages from the moment of birth, and that these three stages centred upon these three areas of the body respectively.

In the newly born baby, Freud saw the libidinous or 'id' instinct (see page 44) as a turbulent mass of ungoverned desire, searching for and demanding gratification while lacking the means of rationalizing the best approach to gaining it. In a just-born infant Freud saw this drive as inhabiting the entire body of the infant, investing internal organs, musculature and skin alike. This phase is immediately superseded by the beginning of the oral period in which the organ of primary importance to sexual gratification is the mouth, for instance in being breast-fed. The oral period is regarded as lasting from birth to the end of the first year of life.

The breast becomes associated in the baby's mind at a very early stage with love, security and nourishment, and so, by that token, with Mother, who provides these necessities. The manner in which security is first threatened, is when the infant becomes aware of the sexual nature of the Father. The earliest love for a person other than 'self', is for Mother, and this love is in no sense sexual in today's use of the term but it does possess an erotic element and that is held responsible for girls having a harder emotional adjustment to make in their early development than boys. For if you are a girl your first love in life is for a person of the same sex as yourself, whereas a boy loves for the first time someone of the opposite sex.

A Baby Boy's Development

You might suppose on the strength of this observation, that a boy's development to puberty and manhood would be perfectly straightforward emotionally, and that love for Mother would develop and flower, and gradually come to bear the fruit of mature love for girlfriend or lover. This mode of development would be ideal in every sense, for it would represent a smooth traversing of the entire spectrum of instinctive feeling from love of Mother as supplier of nourishment and security (necessary for self-preservation), merging into a love first and foremost erotic but containing a vestige of the instinctual need for self-preservation.

What happens, though, is rather different. As the earliest sexuality extends to show a little boy's Mother as a woman, so also it extends to reveal Father as a man. The baby then feels very strongly that he is rivalling Father for the love of Mother, and powerful undercurrents of hatred, jealousy, anxiety and guilt arise, bringing with them intense conflict. Because he hates his Father he feels guilty, and fears also that he may be deprived of his Mother's love and nourishment, since Father is obviously the stronger of the two. This makes him feel extremely insecure.

Father, then, is a distinct obstacle to self-preservation. And if the baby boy continues to love his Mother as he did before the realization dawned on him, he fears the loss of the elements necessary for self-preservation. To cease to love Mother erotically, however, is to deny the strength of the recently engendered sex drive, and that seems to the child an equally intolerable outcome. He is therefore caught in a conflict between the need for self-preservation, and the need for sexual gratification.

A Baby Girl's Development

The situation which the baby girl faces arises when she first perceives Father as 'man' and 'male', and she is both scared and fascinated at the idea of loving him, for the prospect is both stimulating and perilous. Supposing her instincts bid her love her Father; might this not lose her the love of her Mother, and so cut her off from the supply of love, nourishment and security that she needs? Again, to deny the awakening desire to make Father an erotic love-object, is to deny an instinct different from, but equal in strength to, the self-preservation urge. So the baby girl, like the baby boy, is in a state of conflict, for to seek gratification of one primal need appears automatically to cut her off from gratification of the other.

As we will see later, people who cope unsuccessfully with conflicts arising at the oral stage of their development, sometimes called 'oral personalities', tend either to be supremely and gloriously happy, or abysmally unhappy. This is related to the fact that, during the oral phase, when the 'id' still reigns supreme and there is neither 'ego' nor 'super-ego' to reason and to compromise, the young child tends to react with the 'all or nothing' response. A small baby is either totally contented, for example when he is being cuddled and/or fed by his parents, or wildly unhappy with a deep and untempered grief when he lacks these things.

In the course of normal development the child passes unscathed through the 'all or nothing' phase, although of course, if the oral conflicts remain unresolved they will manifest themselves in another form later on. Babies of either sex have in reality to choose between Mother and Father — neither hating nor loving Father will actually deprive the child of its Mother and all that she symbolizes. But the important thing, is that this is how it appears on the surface to the infantile mind, the true conflict meanwhile going on internally and at a much deeper level. The conflict is of course between the two great basic instincts, of self-preservation and sex.

Worry and Conflict

This serves to illustrate the difference, in hypnotherapists' language, between *worry* and *conflict*. *Worry* is present in the conscious mind, and something one is aware of; or, as we can say in the case of the baby, what appears to it to be a battle to keep Mother and either love or rival Father, is *worry*. The *conflict* refers to the struggle taking place within, i.e., in the subconscious mind where primeval instincts are stored.

Since all babies face these conflicts, why are they not all injured by them? The majority of us, thankfully, develop normally, by resolving the conflicts with the help of a secure background and plenty of parental love. Early conflicts of this type, however, lay the foundations for the development of schizoid problems later in life.

Gratification and Anger

There are other conflicts to contend with during the oral phase. In the early stages, gratification, pleasure and satisfaction are gained from breast feeding and sucking. The intensity of the satisfaction obtained, is equivalent in baby terms to sexual desire rewarded with sexual gratification, and as the baby has not yet learned to relate to his environment properly, nor learned that interruptions of pleasure are inevitable, interference with his gratification brings on intense anger and resentment on his part.

You may be breast or bottle feeding a baby who is obviously thoroughly enjoying the process. The doorbell rings, and you place him carefully in his cot while you go to answer the door. Almost inevitably the child will scream at the interruption of his feed. You think that this is because he is hungry, and he may well be. Life must go on — and small babies learn that the entire world does not revolve around them.

Self-Directed Rage

But unless a frustrated and angry child is shown plenty of love and understanding, and made above all to feel appreciated and wanted, the violent rage he experiences whenever his pleasure is interrupted *will be directed inwardly at himself;* and this is productive of a great deal of self-frustration and self-blame. This happens because the baby is unaware of anything (other than parents) outside himself, and has no concept of an environment capable of interfering with his own particular source of pleasure.

Normally an older child or adult can 'apportion blame', i.e., identify the cause of a personal disturbance, and realize that he/she is not to blame for it.

Anger may be directed in such a circumstance at the event or the object or person responsible for frustrated gratification, but anger and rage and scorn would not be inwardly directed. A baby directs his anger at himself for he knows no better. If this pattern is allowed to develop into a habit and the child's pleasure is frequently whipped away from it without explanation or a comforting cuddle, then a conditioned response is set up in the infant's and child's mind, known as 'rage turned inwards'. This, psychologically speaking, is an unhealthy state of affairs, and can predispose to the development of depressive illness later in life.

Dissociation
Unfortunately in some ways, a frustrated infant has an alternative method of coping with frustration. He can retreat within himself, and refuse to experience pleasure and gratification by 'dissociating' in his own mind the activity such as feeding at the breast that gives him such intense pleasure, from the pleasure itself. Actions from that point onwards become 'stereotyped' and 'mechanical', and devoid of feeling. The sense of gratification which, as we have seen, embodies the baby's expression of his sexual instinct, is repressed. It remains locked within the subconscious mind for perhaps a number of years, ultimately emerging in the form of a schizoid personality or even frank schizophrenia.

All that I have written so far about the development of various psychological conditions is 'general' and rather simplistically explained. This book is about hypnotherapy and the kind of problems with which it can deal, and in order to understand, for example, how hypnotherapy can be of benefit to a depressed person, or to someone suffering from a phobia, it is necessary to understand what depression and phobias are and in what ways the mind is disturbed when they are present. So don't fall into the trap of thinking that every time your child cries he is developing 'rage turned inwards' — or that when the girl baby refuses to smile at either parent then she is being overwhelmed with primal conflicts between sexual desire and the need for self-preservation!

What she has probably got, is a touch of colic or 'the moodies' and nothing to worry about at all. It is essential to preserve a strict sense of proportion when writing and reading about these mental and emotional disorders, and there is no earthly reason to suppose suddenly that you, or your children, are developing some awful neurotic illness. Nevertheless, this brief account should give you some idea of how mental illness is engendered in early life.

Returning to the baby who learns to 'dissociate' his or her emotions from gratifying activities — if the 'all or nothing' response has developed earlier during its oral phase, the extent to which it represses emotion will be emphasized, and the ultimate symptoms he or she experiences will be all the more severe. Conversely, if the young child does *not* 'dissociate' the experience of pleasure from pleasurable activity, the 'all or nothing' response makes depressive illnes all the more likely to develop!

The experiences a baby has, either of love and security or of unresolved conflict, during his first year of life, produce feelings that predispose it to one sort of outlook on life and behaviour rather than another, as an older child and as an adult. Each one of us is an individual and hence perceives and interprets events accordingly. No two children will grow up identically with respect to behaviour and temperament regardless of the similarity of their surroundings; but the early oral conflicts and how these are handled, or left to cause trouble, predispose a child very much towards a particular form of behaviour, and towards mental health or lack of it.

An infant deprived of Mother's love, will grow up with a feeling of deprivation no matter what its later experiences or relationships. Deprivation of this type, causes inhibition and conditioning which helps to create the predisposition towards a particular neurotic condition or set of physical symptoms. The man or woman who derives most joy from life, is the one who has developed fewest inhibitions and has been least deprived as an infant.

Compulsive Traits

The subtle and complex patterns which form within us during our oral phase, remain with us all our lives. And there is a further manner in which early (oral) conflicts can affect us. Among other things, early conflicts of the kind we have been discussing here, create inner tension of which neither depression nor schizoid traits need be the result. If the tension is very severe, *some kind of compulsive activity* is indulged in later in life, as a means of releasing tension. This sets up a habit pattern, and is a common reason for hypnotherapy consultations, for the compulsive act is generally annoying and upsetting to the person concerned and may even earn him a certain amount of ridicule from family or colleagues at work if his habit is observed.

The person experiences an overwhelming temptation to carry out some particular action over and over again — for instance, turning off light switches and taps, and returning time and time again to see that they are all switched off, despite the knowledge that this is so. The effort involved, always far outweighs the value of the act in itself, and driven on by a power he is unaware of in his subconscious, the victim of compulsive activity is obliged to repeat the action again and again.

If he is prevented from his compulsive acts, the individual knows no peace, but experiences anger and intense anxiety until allowed to return to his usual habit. If he tries to give up the habit of his own volition, then he feels profoundly depressed until he gives in and recommences his compulsive acts.

On achieving his goal, the poor victim derives no true satisfaction from it — he experiences a temporary release from tension and then the pattern restarts. Essentially there exists at the bottom of this puzzling illness, an unreasoning and compelling drive before which the person is powerless. For although the goal in view may be a reasonable one, for instance housework, the urge to complete it is pursued with such vigour and to the neglect of so many other considerations, that the effect is startling. This is an example of the 'all or nothing' reaction coming into play.

People whose oral conflicts have never been satisfactorily resolved, tend to be shy and insecure, and subject to self-doubt. Their ride through life is generally a rough one, for the slightest word of criticism from lover, close friend or family sends them into a decline of intense self-doubt, for they react to what they construe as disapproval in a very exaggerated way. They are so very easily hurt that they are correspondingly terrified of hurting other people, and are unable to do so, or even to show a sign of aggression when the occasion demands, for this reaction hurts them even more. This is why they are often the victim of bullies and aggressive people at work or among the family members.

Depressive Illness

Their position in life is basically a self-destructive one, and this is never more fully realized than when they develop *depressive illness*. People suffering from this form of neurosis, feel at times extremely ill and occasionally fail to receive the love, support and comfort they need because their friends and family are too accustomed to their overreacting and taking every little blow to heart. They are frequently riddled with self-doubt and self-abnegation and it is nothing new to those around them who may well miss the fact that depressive illness is the diagnosis, and treatment speedily required.

The depressed person has to contend with both physical and mental symptoms, and their combined effect can make life extremely hard to bear — so hard, in fact, that suicide is a rising statistic among people suffering from this illness. Emotionally he feels a strange combination of 'numbness' or a total vacuity of feeling, while at the same time being aware of overwhelming hopelessness, despair and irretrievable loss. Depressive illness may come on for no apparent reason, in which case it is known as 'endogenous' (coming from within), or it may be precipitated by a set of circumstances in the external environment, job loss, redundancy, a bereavement, for example.

When there are apparent reasons for the person feeling as he does, for example after the death of a loved one, the intense emotional grief is considered normal and we term it mourning. When the sadness and desire to withdraw, are out of all proportion to the precipitating cause, and the bereavement reaction goes on and on, then the person is said to be suffering from exogenous depression (depression precipitated by an external event) or, if very prolonged, then from melancholia.

Subjectively, the man, woman or (rarely) child, feels inert, withdrawn, purposeless and at their lowest ebb. They have no wish, no desire, no energy and no motivation whatever for continuing to live. Some depressed people sit around or lie in bed for days on end, too sick and too little motivated even to try to end their own lives. The risk of suicide in this group must never be underestimated, however. It is not true to say that because a person mentions ideas of killing himself, that he or she would never do so. This is a myth and an unfortunate one, for it is possible that many depressed people would be alive and well today, if their cry for help had been listened to. All very depressed people, whether they discuss suicide or not, are at a potential risk of killing themselves.

If guilt is a predominant feature, and there are concomitant symptoms of restlessness, self-accusation and attempts at self-injury, which at the subconscious level are aimed at atoning for a crime, then the state is referred to as 'agitated melancholia'.

It is worth remembering that any well-balanced person *can* break down if the precipitating circumstances are sufficiently severe. Conversely, a highly abnormal person may never show a sign or symptom of psychological abnormality if life is always 'kind' to him and he is never pushed beyond the boundaries of his own narrow limits.

Schizoid Personality

Before we end this survey of the psychological abnormalities that can result from oral stage conflicts, and go on to look at case histories illustrating these illnesses, we must pay a little attention to the *schizoid personality*. As we saw, schizoid tendencies gain their first chance to germinate when there is a failure to resolve the very early dilemma of 'loving father/possibly losing mother' in the case of a baby girl, or of 'loving mother/hating father who may remove mother from me', in the case of a boy baby. These tendencies gain a further hold over the personality later in the oral stage, if there is 'rage turned inward' which is not resolved, but dealt with by the infant 'dissociating' action and pleasure.

People with schizoid personalities are reserved, shy and retiring, and tend to be what Jung called 'introverted'. They are far too concerned about their own personal feelings on a subject and how they react to a given situation, to pay much attention to objective observation. Not necessarily selfish, they are very self-centred in the sense that they are the very centre of their own universe. They take things extremely seriously because they have 'inner values' that other people are unaware of, as well as a rich fantasy life and a pronounced tendency to build castles in the air. When the castles appear air-borne to them, all is well; but when the obviously inadequate foundations become apparent they react with intense misery, disappointment and disillusionment.

Schizoid people often have a strongly creative urge, and many artists, writers, poets and painters have had this type of personality. They are typically very frustrated until they find a medium for expressing their creativity. This applies equally well to their emotional life, for they are capable of tremendous depths of feeling, but are often cruelly incapable of expressing them.

Schizoid people also illustrate the 'all or nothing' response, because they are either bright, euphoric and joyous — or intensely and deeply depressed. They are rarely aggressive, they blame themselves when things go wrong, and fear hurting others to the point of being unable to defend themselves when necessary. They are grossly oversensitive, and have an overdeveloped sense of tragedy coupled with an enormous capacity for suffering.

Schizoid people prefer to live in the past, because they attach enormous importance to happy memories and because they have an innate fear that the present and the future will be disappointing to them. Although they lack worldly wisdom, the ability to appreciate materialistic viewspoints etc., they make up for it with a highly developed intuition and an inherent ability to interpret dreams and symbols occurring in the life of others. One of the chief obstacles in their relationships with other people is the fact that they feel unable to communicate adequately. Their values, feelings, meanings and intuitions, although perfectly clear to them within their own minds, are very difficult to relate to others however close they would like to be to them.

There follows some case history accounts of patients who have requested hypnotherapy for their problems, the diagnosis made in each case, and the treatment carried out.

5. Case Histories of the Oral Types

The following case histories are taken from files containing the personal details of real patients with very real problems. The details of the development of symptoms and the history of the psychological illness in each case are true to life; but I have altered details pertaining to personal identity in order that the patient's right to confidentiality and privacy should be observed at all times.

Depression (1)

Anne L. came to see me shortly after I started to see hypnotherapy patients, and the symptoms of which she complained were those of classic depression. She even told me the diagnosis — which is not unusual these days, when people are much better informed than they used to be and the symptomatology of illnesses such as depression and anxiety are well known.

I don't just mean that Anne came to me and told me that she was depressed! Anyone could do that, without even really knowing the meaning of the word. No, Anne was a University graduate with a first class honours degree in psychology — and there was no doubt in her mind that depression was the name of her complaint, despite the fact that she had so far been unable to do anything to help herself. There was no doubt in my mind, either, that she was right — after I had heard her story. These are the essential details:

She was twenty-one years old, and had graduated the previous summer in psychology at London University. She came from a single parent family and had three much younger brothers — and a hard-working mother who was deputy headmistress now of Anne's old school. Her father had left home when she, Anne, was just eleven — and consequently she had had to play 'mother' to her younger brothers for some years, coping in the evening and the early morning and taking over to allow her mother to pursue her teaching career. Anne had never resented this, and in fact had always enjoyed an excellent relationship with her mother. Her father she was less open about — she simply volunteered that he was 'a brilliant man, and very critical' of his children.

She, Anne, had been well and fairly happy and had won a scholarship to University where she had done extremely well. She had never known the meaning of the word depression until three months after Finals when she broke off with her boyfriend whom she had discovered to be two-timing her. A few days after that, she had felt 'strange', inert, very fatigued and quite soon, despairing — and had come to seek advice from me in preference to seeing a psychiatrist as she feared 'simply being told to take pills'.

I thought the combined effects of examination strain and breaking up with her boyfriend had precipitated her attack of depression, which was relatively straightforward, with such characteristic features as poor sleeping, especially at night when trying to fall asleep; poor appetite; extreme physical and mental inertia; preoccupations with death; and periods of uncontrollable weeping. But I looked for an underlying cause in the oral phase of her development, the point of origin of most depression. And I discovered that the marriage between Anne's mother and father had been most strained during the eighteen months after she was born.

It seemed that — as Anne remembered under trance conditions — that her father had disliked his wife breast-feeding Anne in front of him — and whenever this had occurred, he had started to rage and shout, necessitating his wife returning the baby to her cot and attending to him. Consequently, the number of occasions on which Anne had inadvertently experienced 'rage turned inwards' when her breast sucking pleasure was interrupted, were innumerable. The feeling of inadequacy and guilt at the time, had been reinforced by the sounds of her father shouting abuse in the background — which she as a baby had interpreted as further evidence of her own worthlessness.

We reached this memory quite easily in the second session, by my using a 'regression' technique, i.e., under conditions of a hypnotic trance, suggesting to my patient that she turn back the pages of a book containing the detailed story of her life. We went back year after year quite uneventfully until the time Anne was two months — it was then her subconscious mind was able to 'remember' the details of the traumatic breastfeeding instances that had laid the seed for her self-directed rage and doubt.

I gave Anne some ego-boosting treatment after she had remembered the traumatic period adequately, and had shed some tears about it. I suggested that her confidence was getting greater daily and that the upsetting scenes in her infancy that had bothered her so much — were evidence of her father's inability to cope with being a father, not with her inadequacy as a daughter or person. And I used what is known as 'ideomotor signalling' — I got Anne into a deep state of trance then asked her to reply to me with a 'yes' or 'no' signal, by moving the forefinger of her right hand.

Once I was certain we were communicating, I told her to pump her finger up and down, this being the symbol for ridding her system of bad feelings about her father which her subconscious had harboured for twenty years. Vigorous pumping resulted from my commands and after two such sessions of getting rid of the effects of a bullying parent, Anne's depression started to clear. She needed in all about six further ego-boosting sessions, before she felt she was sufficiently recovered to manage alone.

Depression (2)
Another depressed patient who came to me for advice and treatment, was a sixty-five year old chauffeur who had retired two months previously. He was complaining of inability to sleep at night; lack of interest in his usual hobbies of photography and golf; and extreme irritability with his wife and daughter. Again, like Anne L. he had had no similar trouble until the day he retired — by which I mean he had no previous history of mental illness or depression. Certainly Joe P. had had a life of tension — who would not, driving in the London traffic at the beck and call of a moody millionaire? — but never before had he experienced such devastating feelings of worthlessness and despair.

The first time I put Joe into a trance, I suggested that in his imagination he was lying on a warm sandy beach by a beautiful blue sea. I told him he had everything around him he could wish for . . . and before I could proceed with my suggestion technique he had burst into tears. Although still in a state of mild trance

Joe was able to tell me that what he did not have around him was his working gear — chauffeur's uniform, chamois leather, duster! Far from finding a sunny beach a delightful place to be in, he had broken down as the memory of his compulsory retirement came to him. All that was wrong with Joe — was reactive depression consequent upon his having to retire, and all he wanted was to return to work!

I gave some calming and confidence-boosting suggestions to Joe when he was next in a condition relaxed enough to receive them (it was during the following session together); in addition, I made some practical suggestions to him on an ordinary conversational basis, as to where to look for a part-time driving job. He was very keen on the idea and rang me a week later, over the moon because he had found himself fifteen hours of freelance driving per week.

Joe's type of depression was fairly clearly the reactive type. I am sure that had we spent hours in extensive analysis I could have discovered an oral conflict responsible for his tendency to become depressed. But there would have been no particular point in this. He had reacted badly, as so many fit older men do, to being 'put out to grass' as he termed it, and as soon as we had pinpointed the problem and found a possible solution his symptoms cleared up at once.

Compulsive Trait (1)

Here is an example of a patient who came to consult me because he wished to get rid of a compulsive habit that had troubled him for three years. Alan A. was an insurance broker in Central London, aged about thirty-eight, and with all the appurtenances of a successful and 'with it' business executive, from smart company car to expense account lunches and adoring secretaries. But the poor man was wretched! Alan was in fact an old friend of my husband — we had both known him for years; so he was able to come to the point quite easily with us.

'I don't know how to tell you this, Caroline', he said, obviously embarrassed; 'I've started this ridiculous practice — I don't know how to tell you — and I'm terrified someone will find out!'

He was under a certain amount of strain at the time, approaching the end of his study course with the Open University, and in addition had recently been told that his father was suffering from inoperable cancer. One evening, after a particularly busy day, he had suddenly had the urge to scrub out the loo! Fortunately he was at home at the time and had merely cleaned it and had a bath and gone to bed. Since then, however, (some two months in all) he had felt compelled to scrub the loo really hard each morning before leaving home, and had twice made himself late in so doing.

Once he had refused to give in to what he considered to be an absurd urge, and had felt out of sorts and tense all day. He admitted that when he had completed the job, he felt 'relaxed, tranquil and peaceful' — but was not in that state for long before the urge started to bother him again. He was quite besides himself with anxiety when he came to see me — for that very day he had felt a similar compulsion to clean out the loo at work!

Alan could think of no reason whatever why this should all have come about. He then admitted that he had had a 'bout' of similar trouble three years previously but it had died a natural death, for it had coincided with a severe row he had had with a girlfriend, and had disappeared when they got together again. It now seemed that he and Mary had parted finally, and that he was missing her and consequently this added to his present sum of strain.

I took him back in stages of regression, with no result before the age of two years. He was able to 'see' with his subconscious memory, and recount to me a time when his mother had been changing him in the bathroom and powdering him after a warm bath. It seemed that the telephone rang and his mother put him down on the loo which she was in the process of flushing — and that he had laid there cold and crying while she answered the telephone. The noise of the water frightened him and when his mother had returned, she had told him that if he was naughty again (i.e., persisted in screaming) she would flush him away down the loo — and had held him over it to scare him!

He had had a fair amount of maternal love during the crucial stages of his development — but obviously not enough, for he had never quite resolved the conflict in his mind about Mummy's and Daddy's love. It was apparent from something he said, that he had equated being punished by a flushing loo, with being wicked enough to love mummy and rival daddy; although his conscious mind did not remember this at all.

I treated Alan by improving his confidence and lessening his tension by means of suggesting, under light trance, that he would grow more and more sure of himself, less and less affected by tension, and feel less and less frequently the compulsion to loo clean. And I planted a post-hypnotic suggestion, that whenever he felt an uncontrollable urge to do so at home — he would count to three slowly, feel peace flowing into him, and either make himself a cup of tea or take the dog for a walk, depending on the time of day. I also suggested that if the urge should come over him while he was at work or elsewhere away from home, he would be able to help himself by a deep breathing technique I taught him.

He fell prey to the compulsion once more at home — after an upsetting telephone call; but no more at work. Gradually his confidence became adequate to enable him to deal with the fear of the compulsion, and I got him to 'pump out' his negative feelings about lavatories and the infantile threat of punishment. In two months he had got over the problem altogether.

Compulsive Trait (2)
The next case of compulsive action, was also successful, and it makes a good example of the kind of case any hypnotherapist may come across any day of the week.

Janet M. was recommended to me by a friend of hers whom I had been treating for obesity. She was a pleasant forty-year-old secretary with a responsible job in the Company for whom she had worked for eleven years. Her complaint was as follows:

'I've often had funny little habits, and as a child I can remember avoiding the lines between the paving stones, having to check each toy three times before I shut the play cupboard door, things like that.

'I've always managed to cope, but just recently I've started to count all the coins in my purse and subdivide them into copper and silver in the different compartments. I feel absolutely "obliged" to do this, for some unknown reason, and it's very inconvenient on the bus going to and from work, because sometimes of course in the rush hour I don't get a seat, and if I am standing up to count them I tend to drop them . . . then they have to be counted and sorted all over again!'

I was able to tell at once that the habit was more than 'inconvenient' to her, it was making her life a misery, especially since she was scared that colleagues from work who used the same bus route, might see her counting her money compulsively.

I took a case history from her, noting details of her early life, relationship with parents and so on; and I explained to her that her compulsive habit had arisen as a means of coping with anxiety and tension caused by unresolved conflict during her first year or so of life. She looked a bit incredulous at this statement, as patients often do when such a thing is pointed out to them. And I did not have even to place her in a trance state, for her to be able to recall the very events in her life which surely did the damage to her young psyche. And to clinch my suspicions that her problem was a compulsive one, I asked her whether she felt depressed if she attempted to avoid the counting and temporarily relieved when she had performed the act; both answers were in the affirmative.

Her early childhood trauma had been inflicted by her mother leaving home, baby and husband when she, Janet, was only three months old; the rest of her childhood she spent with her father, and a succession of 'lady friends', none of whom she had liked or really got to know.

This lifestyle had been quite sufficient to engender unresolved conflict and inner tension which was obliged to find an outlet later in life. She was a good hypnotic subject and I was able to suggest to her that compulsive behaviour would trouble her less and less now that she knew the reason for its having affected her; that she was a capable, efficient, pleasant and worthwhile person who had every reason to feel proud of herself and her achievements in life, and that all tendencies to count objects — coins or otherwise — would cease to bother her.

She additionally helped herself by taking up Yoga and in so doing, learned how to relax thoroughly and to use breathing techniques to instil a feeling of confidence and tranquillity. Our combined efforts overcame the problem for her, within about four weeks of her first consultation.

Schizoid Personality
Andrew P., a thirty-three-year-old clerk, is an obvious example among my past patients to use in illustrating schizoid personality. He came to see me after being persuaded to do so by his girl-friend to whom he was fairly closely attached considering that people of this type do not easily form close relationships, as I pointed out above.

He had, in fact, had a succession of girl-friends, none of whom had understood him at all, or so he informed me. I personally think that they probably got to know him too well and felt that they could not handle him; for he was an unusual mixture of the shy and the retiring, while also appearing to have a terrible grudge against the world for not appreciating his musical talents. He had been to College to study music, but had reacted so vehemently to any criticism offered of his work by his tutors that two terms there made the Principal decide that Andrew and a music degree course were incompatible.

He alternated now, so his girl-friend told me, between building fantastic plans that quite obviously would never materialize — such as the two of them travelling around the world as buskers, performing in the streets by singing and playing musical instruments whenever they needed money — and experiencing tremendous disappointment and disillusionment when she pointed out to him the impracticality of his ideas. However, not only was he good looking and often generous, but she (Maureen) felt a sympathy for him and had stayed with him longer than previous lovers.

I did not say to Andrew in so many words: 'You have a schizoid personality' — as I might have told a patient that they were suffering from depression or an anxiety neurosis, but I confirmed that I thought he had some deep-rooted difficulties to face and overcome, and asked detailed questions during our first consultation about his early childhood and his parents.

Apart from the fact that he admitted that he had not liked his father (who was now dead) and that he did not think his mother had been very friendly towards him and his brother, he could say nothing else. *Hypnoanalysis* seemed to be the best solution so I explained to him what it involved, and for the next week I saw him daily for one hour, getting rid of his fears and misconceptions about hypnotism and generally teaching him how to be as susceptible as possible to hypnosis. At the end of that time, he was able to enter the trance state immediately I suggested that he would; carry out post-hypnotic suggestions quickly and easily; and remember with ease, various scenes and places. He could do this in two different ways — he could *regress*, i.e., go back to a place or situation, but view it from his present point of view; and *revivify*, i.e., go back in his mind and actually relive the event.

The next stage was to utilize the psychoanalytic technique of free association, and get him to start with a random word or idea, and say the various things each successive word suggested to him. We had a number of hours spent like this and whenever he showed any resistance we resorted to 'hypnotic recall'. This means that I would straight away put him in a trance and so discover the nature of the material his conscious mind was anxious to avoid referring to. I got him to 'regress' at this stage, as he was not yet ready to relive his experience.

The result was that, although resistance to free association was present, my using hypnotic recall in this way caused him to re-enact the causative traumatic event in his babyhood when in a state of trance. Shortly after this, the same material to which resistance had formerly been shown, appeared in the waking state during a free association session. This happens because the process of revelation under hypnosis, boosts the conscious ego, and strengthens and prepares it to accept the painful facts disclosed under trance conditions.

The injurious experience Andrew had gone through, causing the development of his schizoid personality had been the total denial of mother's love on a number of occasions between the ages of one and three years. Andrew's brother Peter had been born one year after Andrew, and this had given his mother severe post-natal depression, judging by what he could recall of her withdrawn behaviour after Peter's birth. Andrew could, under hypnosis, actually recall going up to her as a toddler just learning to walk and to speak, and climbing on to her knee to cuddle her. She would just push him away, and tell him not to be such a nuisance.

I did not cause Andrew to relive the unhappy memories in real life, i.e., in the waking state, until I was certain that all the relevant material had come to light. Various details had to be tied up so that I was sure that we could evoke memories of sufficient significance to cause a genuine *abreaction* when the time came — i.e., the reliving of the events with the accompanying appropriate emotion, which is an effective way of getting rid of repressed anger and the 'rage that is turned inwards' when basic emotional needs are denied or continually interfered with.

The fact that Andrew's mother pushed him away and told him he was bothering her, made him blame himself and rage inwardly at the self that was so undesirable and so unlovable that he did not win even his mother's affection.

Having caused Andrew to abreact in the waking state when I felt he was ready to do so, and having released a tremendous amount of pent-up anger, grief and self-loathing, the final phase of the procedure was entered upon. This consisted of 're-educating' him to dispel the false ideas, standards, attitudes and goals that he had accumulated over the years, originating in misconceptions, misinterpretations and a need to erect a barrier of defence. What this amounts to in fact, is the rearranging of the personality upon sounder foundations and along healthier lines than the fragile structure previously supporting it.

It was not sufficient merely to talk this over with Andrew, who was already beginning to feel a different person, and get him to agree that he would think differently. Suggestions have to be made along re-educational lines to the subconscious mind of the person and they have to be reinforced with post-hypnotic suggestions. I suggested to Andrew, for example, that he would try again for a place in College to study music as he was certainly gifted and wished to do so very much. I also boosted his ego, increasing his confidence and making him happy with his new, properly functioning self.

I am pleased to say that he responded very well to this dynamic investigation of his personality, the abreaction (although it was a painful experience), and the aftercare of positive suggestions and therapy to boost the ego. He succeeded in his now realistic ambition, because he was able to comprehend the nature of criticism and to accept it. And far from continuing to build castles in the air, he became a more realistic person — and was happily married to Maureen last time I heard of him.

The schizoid personality is one of several psychopathologies that respond to hypnoanalysis; others include hysterical conversion syndrome, alcoholism, kleptomania, frigidity and symptomatic asthma. Not every one of these is cured every single time by hypnoanalysis; but success is permanent if the technique is effective and it serves a tremendously useful purpose in the range of hypnotic techniques available for therapy.

6. Anal Conflicts

As we saw in Chapter 4, the second important stage in a child's life is the 'anal stage'. This stage begins shortly before the end of the first year of the child's life and lasts approximately until the age of three. Of course, there is no clear-cut division between the oral stage and the anal stage — they overlap and run concurrently for a little, until oral phase characteristics merge gradually and imperceptibly into anal phase ones.

It is called the 'anal' stage because it is considered that its hallmark is the child's aim to expel (i.e., open his bowels) aggressively, and later to retain his motions, at his own will; he becomes able to do this, once he has gained control of his 'anal sphincter', the circular band of muscle at the outlet of the rectum, which can be relaxed or constricted at will, whenever a bowel movement is to be expelled or contained. It was, according to Freud, also the area of sexual significance during the time we are discussing.

The small child also becomes aware of himself as increasingly separate from his mother and from those who supply his needs. He is, in fact, beginning to develop his own identity, and during this time the basic essentials of child-parents relationship are laid as the child learns to distinguish between the 'me' and the 'not me'. For he is learning that he must relate not only to his parents but also to the environment around him. Whereas before, he had an intense need to focus on the breast, he now has an equally strong need to focus upon bowel control.

Naturally there will be battles with Mother over this. Compliance with her wishes regarding bowel control, brings reward and praise, and non-compliance tends to bring disapproval and possibly punishment. From the child's point of view there is here a combination of circumstances just as enraging

and frustrating as denial of the breast during the oral stage. He
has to learn to adapt to withdrawal of the breast as a source of
nourishment, and in this way some distancing between himself
and his Mother. Together with withdrawal of the breast, goes
withdrawal of the warmth and intimacy that is associated with
breast-feeding.

In addition to this, the struggle to master bowel control can
at times lead to confrontations between child and Mother, and
the apparent withdrawal of love. The little boy or girl also starts
to learn that reward and punishment are associated with success
and failure in controlling his bowel function. Battles over toilet-
training are also likely to be followed by battles over eating,
dressing and so on, together with other activities as the child begins
to exert his own ego. Often the child may display an unusual
spirit of contrariness, when he learns to exert his own will. The
child also discovers that he can, in fact, by using his will, obtain
gratifying results, by being obliging, by pleading, and even
sometimes by subterfuge.

At the same time all of this is going on, the child is learning
how to talk and how to use his mind. Exploration of his immediate
environment becomes a fascinating study. And at the same time,
he is also gaining mastery over his ability to move about. All
sorts of stimuli make themselves felt. The child learns that unless
he is careful he can fall downstairs, that fires burn, that some
things have to be approached with caution and others do not,
that some things may be touched and others may not be touched.

He observes that when some objects fall to the ground, they
break — and that when others fall, they do not break; that it
is permissible to play with a rubber ball, but that it is not
permissible to throw one of Mother's best china teacups on the
floor! Thus a system of wider responses is developing; instead
of there just being reciprocal communication between Mother
and child, or between breast and mouth, there are responses to
the all-important business of toilet training, to learning how to
dress, how to eat unaided, how to walk, how to get one's own
way, and how to react to reward and punishment. The world
has become a very much larger place, and the child begins to
learn how to master his environment.

The problem of learning rudimentary self-control, not only
over one's physical functions such as going to the toilet, crawling
and walking, but also over one's emotions, has begun. The child

now discovers that rage is not always productive, and that crying does not always produce the results that he wants, just as he finds that by certain kinds of behaviour he can obtain the pleasure and approval he needs. He also finds that he can in fact be very upsetting to his parents, and particularly to his Mother. Consequently, he even begins to learn that he can inflict pain on others, although at this time of course he does not have sufficient awareness to appreciate the depths or quality of suffering that he may cause.

Ano-Sadistic Period

As a result there is often a sadistic element to the influence he forms in his mind, which is why, in classical psychology, the anal period is sometimes called the ano-sadistic period. However, although the small child is starting to separate from his Mother and to develop his own identity, we must not make the mistake of believing that the infant is any the less attached to her. In fact, the period from nine months to three years, is thought to be the time of greatest attachment, for the child is still to a considerable extent very dependent upon the Mother, not only for love and the security which that brings, but also for food and for locomotion.

Furthermore, the child is very much engrossed with exploring his environment, and is therefore subject to all kinds of dangers, so the Mother assumes considerable importance in the role of 'protectress'. She can generally be relied upon to appear when the child cries for help, and is a constant buffer, physically and emotionally, between the developing youngster and the mistakes he makes in the course of his early explorations. Burned fingers, electrical shocks, grazed knees and bumped heads, not to mention a scratch from a teased cat or nip from a dog who dislikes having his tail pulled — all come as unpleasant surprises to the young toddler who until recently has been protected from the indifferent universe by his devoted parents. Now Mother is, in some ways, even more important — she renews his frequently shattered sense of security and repairs his loss of dignity — something young children paradoxically have without being aware of the fact until it is temporarily disturbed.

In this way, the Mother is both helping the child, and training him to cope with the many dangers of his immediate environment. Besides being there to care and console, she is also there to correct and if necessary to punish; so although the child is beginning to assume a separate identity and is becoming aware of people and relationships, hazards and obligations, he is still essentially dependent for love and security upon his Mother. Thus separation from the Mother at this stage, for whatever reason, can be the source of considerable difficulties later on in the child's life when he is adult, and productive of much insecurity and many difficulties in relating to other people through lack of trust.

Equally traumatic to a young child and equally capable of inflicting injuries that will maim his psychological development, can be the attitude of the parents, in particular of the Mother, to him during this time of learning and change. He (or she) may be very aggravating, defiant and disobedient, and if intelligent may learn how to play one parent off against the other, refuse to comply with toilet training, and cry, scream, produce temper tantrums and even appear unwell, in concentrated attempts to assert himself and to get his own way.

Every Mother (and Father) is human, and being so is as subject as her young child to aggression and to feelings of frustration, especially when fatigue, stress and tension play a major role in her life. With perhaps several young children to care for, a full or part-time job, domestic work in the home and, let us suppose, a no more than good-to-middling relationship with her husband, it is not at all surprising that a defiant and soiling toddler can be literally the final straw. Comparatively few mothers actually batter their children, and the resultant severe trauma to the child's mind if he is subject to frequent or even several onslaughts of physical attack, is obvious.

But I am here mentioning the parent or Mother who in many respects is average in her ability to cope, and sometimes comforts her child while at other times she punishes him when he did not really deserve to be punished, or loses patience with him when he was trying to please. The child has to learn that not even his relationship with Mother is always calm and that sometimes he receives less than justice from those he loves. But it is essential to maintain a balance of good and bad (with a great deal more emphasis on the good whenever possible) when dealing with a small child, for the lack of security, and the devastating sensation of betrayal and absence of trust, can seriously warp his emotional and psychological development and lead to a number of maladjustments and states of mental illness.

Classical psychology also traces to this stage, characteristic traits such as possessiveness, stubborness or pronounced independence, which are said to be derived from a child's pleasure in retaining his faeces in the face of parental efforts to train him. Of course, any of these traits carried to extreme, can become pathological — as, also, on the other hand, can the highly desirable characteristics of cleanliness and tidiness. These too, when they become abnormally developed, take on a pathological condition.

According to Freud, the ease or difficulty with which a child passes through the pregenital phases (i.e., the oral and the anal), have considerable influence upon later life. Conflict of a serious and prolonged nature in either of these stages can lead to a fixation of libido in one of those stages — or cause a reversion to one of those stages in later life. Thus in adult life, many basic behavioural attitudes, the feelings of love and hatred, relationships with other people, the ability to both give and receive, respect for authority or defiance of it, together with such mental attitudes as optimism or pessimism, are unconsciously modified by a child's experiences in the pregenital phases.

Anal characteristics such as orderliness, tidiness, thrift, cleanliness and so on, are highly desirable in moderation; even, for example, a certain amount of obstinacy can be very useful at times. It is only when these good and positive qualities become accentuated and extreme, and get out of control, that the subject becomes a 'patient' and suffers from a neurosis.

Three main neurotic types of personality are associated with the anal period. These are the obsessional, the paranoid and the hypochondriacal.

Obsessional People
Obsessional people have an innate drive to control both themselves and their environment. Within reason, of course, this can be a good thing. The research scientist, for example, needs such a drive, together with a capacity for meticulous and painstaking detail (also anal in origin) that often accompanies it. However, when over-emphasized, this type of personality is governed by organization and ritual. They are often fanatically tidy, and in medical science physicians recognize an 'ulcerative colitis' type of personality (clearly an anal and obsessional type, this being even more clearly emphasized by the disease being one

of the large bowel, where faeces are formed).

The typical ulcerative colitis patient has been noted to love arranging things in straight lines, whether the objects are items on a hospital bedside locker or matches taken from a matchbox or knives and forks in a cutlery drawer. He is anxious, tense, ruminative and neither gives nor receives very easily in emotional relationships.

Obsessional people often have a ritual which they carry out on numerous occasions during the day as though they were driven to it by an inner compulsion. This repeated activity is really a defence mechanism invented to prevent some forbidden thought or desire from impinging upon the conscious mind. It comes into operation as a result of unconscious guilt, and the suppressed thought is invariably a disguised form of sexual activity for which the ritual is merely a symbol, or sexual equivalent. Often the obsession with ritual also functions as a mechanism to prevent a feared happening from occurring, and again the cause behind this fear is unconscious guilt.

The ritual is sacrificial/magical, rather like an offering to the gods to avoid their anger and propitiate them for past misdeeds. It is 'hoped' that the ritual will prevent the fear from materializing. Sometimes a ritual may be used to achieve something — in this case it is of purely magical intent, and is habitually carried out in order to make sure that the obsessional will get what he wants. The victim of an obsession is not aware that he is trying to expiate his guilt in this way; the guilt lies buried in his subconscious mind, and all he is aware of is the constant need to repeat again and again some absurd piece of behaviour such as rearranging all the paperclips in a certain pattern on his desk several times a day. He *knows* that this serves no useful purpose, at least so far as his conscious mind is concerned. But he has a great and uncontrollable urge to repeat his particular ritual again and again.

Obviously, predisposition towards this type of behaviour is encouraged by unhealthy bribery by parents when the child is young. The forms that such rituals take are in fact many and varied, and partake of the nature and symbolism of the individual concerned. Some obsessional people, for instance, feel absolutely obliged to avoid treading on the cracks between paving stones; others need to clean their teeth a certain number of times every day; and yet others need to check the front door ten times to see that they have locked it when they have left the house, and, in addition, to have several keys to the same lock hidden about their person as well as a couple under a brick or in a flower pot near to the door, in order to overcome the fear of being locked out! One of the best known and most obvious of rituals is the repetitive washing of hands, and this is often carried out many times a day. Obviously the guilt mechanism is there very apparent, as the washing symbolizes cleansing from sin and guilt. Perhaps the most famous occasion of this type of obsessive activity, is that of Lady Macbeth, washing her hands to free herself from the guilt of Duncan's murder, in Shakespeare's play. Sometimes obsessional ritual is not indulged in as a physical activity but as a mental one. A preoccupation with counting may occur, or there could be a tune, rhyme or phrase that remains in the conscious mind and cannot be disposed of. Often when the obsessional person tries to cease the offending ritual, he discovers in fact that he becomes very much more tense, anxious and worried, and this of course leads him to perform the offending ritual later on when he can stand it no longer. Once that has occurred, he is again much happier and more relaxed, and better able to concentrate.

Obviously when the ritual is not carried out, anxiety mounts up inside the obsessional; and when the ritual is followed this built-up anxiety is released; until the time comes round for the ritual to be performed again. But the innate and subconscious causes are not affected in the slightest and remain, requiring treatment. Some forms of excessive eating and drinking are also due to this type of urge. In the last chapter compulsive activity was discussed, and in some respects obsessional behaviour seems to resemble it. However, there is a very distinct difference between the two.

As we have already remarked, in obsessional behaviour there is always an element of the magical. By 'magical' I mean the type of thinking that conceives of a higher power who demands sacrifices and to whom propitiation is due, with the result that rituals have to be resorted to, which, in some mystical way, serve the purpose and ward off visitations of wrath from avenging gods. This is entirely absent from compulsive activity. Thus the word 'obsessional' usually refers to persistent, repetitive and unwelcome trains of thought, often accompanied by the performance of ritual.

Oral compulsion, on the other hand, consists of impulsions to perform repetitive acts or rituals. Obsessions of recent onset are generally fairly easily eradicated, since the hypnotherapist has only to reduce the patient's general anxiety level through hypnotic relaxation. The obsessional behaviour then disappears, simply because there is no anxiety to produce it. However, when the obsession is a long-standing one it is not sufficient just to reduce the general anxiety, but the undesired thought which is productive of the obsession has also to be dealt with specifically.

There are many obsessional types; they are basically hard working, pay great attention to detail and to their own standing in the community, avoid gossip at all costs, and might be classified as being somewhat submissive, for they will in fact go out of their way to avoid aggression, either by themselves or by others.

Paranoid People

Another type of obsessional (the paranoid individual) is in fact the exact opposite. He is aggressive, suspicious and lacking all regard for the feelings of others. He is basically self-centred and selfish. For him 'might is right' and he is willing to exploit people and ignore their individuality. Although he is extroverted, he is in fact fearful of plots against him; in his view, people are always planning something or other to his detriment. He is vain and boastful, and very possessive; his obsessional characteristics are usually strongly in evidence, in so far as he worships 'the system', and is keen on planning, scheming and controlling.

His strongly materialistic tendencies often enable him to succeed very well in life. He is in his element when playing the game of 'one-upmanship'. Nevertheless he has his own brooding fears, and feels that the rest of the world is ganging up on him intending to harm him. In fact his fears are really the projection of his own plots and schemes against others. He may also take a sadistic pleasure in the abuse of power, and will readily trample upon those weaker than himself, delighting in the process.

He is materialistic, and utilitarian — and always right. Paranoids can of course become highly dangerous, particularly when they fear that others are plotting against them. For instance, a paranoid man walking down the street might well imagine that the person walking innocently behind him is following him with the intent to kill him; and he might well turn round and attack the innocent pedestrian. Hitler is of course the classical example of the paranoid personality. Consequently paranoids are not suitable subjects for hypnotherapy and they require intensive treatment by analytical methods and drug therapy in the psychiatric departments of large hospitals.

Hypochondriacal People

With the last of the anal types of personality, the hypochondriac, the obsessional thoughts are focussed upon some organ or system of the body which is supposedly diseased. The hypochondriac is so absorbed and obsessed with his ailments, he proclaims them to all and sundry, to anybody in fact who will listen and expounds at length upon the pains and the details, some of them quite unpleasant.

His proud preoccupation with his symptoms is in fact the hallmark of this type of person. No-one ever had symptoms to equal his, or a degree of pain to match his degree of pain. Naturally of course there is also a strong element of exhibitionism present, which is a further example of the pride and vanity of anal types.

Usually in fact, hypochondriacs are not suffering from any organic disease and investigations by doctors prove negative. However, sometimes they are even capable of deceiving experienced medical men and undergo operations as a result; these provide plenty of further material for gruesome descriptions and pride in the uniqueness of their illness. No doctor had ever seen such a massive lump/furred-up artery/enormous peptic ulcer — and in their verbal accounts of what took place when the consultant came to see them during a ward round, is usually included an emotional handclasp by the great man himself (or great woman herself), congratulating the patient on bearing so very nobly with such an extreme amount of suffering.

However, although there is nothing organically wrong with hypochondriacs, their pains, symptoms and dysfunctions are as real to them as a broken leg would be to other people. The difference between malingerers, hysterics and hypochondriacs can be expressed adequately as follows: the malingerer may say he has an upset stomach, in order to avoid hard work or responsibility; the hysteric reacts similarly in his subconscious mind and gets a real stomach upset which lacks a physical cause; and the hypochondriac spends his time happily experimenting with new remedies in case he should develop a bad stomach.

The hypnotherapeutic approach to hypochondriasis is to counteract anxiety, and accustom the patient to feeling more relaxed. The result of this is that the increased relaxation, concentration and co-operation enable him to talk more freely about his problems. As a consequence of this, the increased self-objectivity provides the patient with fresh ideas and better understanding of the nature of his symptoms. Sometimes, in suitable patients, a symptom can be 'held on a leash' until the subconscious need for it is understood and ready to be relinquished.

In the following chapter we will have a look at some patients' case histories and at how their anal-phase neuroscs have been treated.

7. Case Histories of the Anal Types

The first case is one of an obsessive-compulsive habit — nailbiting. The patient was a nineteen-year-old fish-shop assistant, called Pollie N., who was very tired of her embarrassing habit and longed to stop it — endeavouring to do so, made her extremely tense and anxious and she had always to return to the habit before the tension mounted to unbearable limits.

Obsessive-Compulsive Personality

Pollie had bitten her nails since a very young age. Her mother had given birth to her at the age of sixteen, and she — Pollie — had been brought up by her grandparents until the age of six. She recounted that she had hated school, where she had been punished at the age of five for soiling herself, and had retained her hatred and dread of schools until she left at sixteen.

She had had constantly recurring dreams of a nightmare type since she was a small child, and these mostly involved waking up in a sweat with the walls closing in on her.

Her mother had married when Pollie was five and she had gone to live with them a year later. Her father was a perfectionist and there were many rows with him. When she came to see me, she tended to lack aggression, even to dislike going out when she could stay at home, but did go out because she hated being alone in the house. She bit her nails whenever she was frightened which was often. She was unable to stop until they were down to a certain level, and said she felt better for a bit when she had a chewing session. She actually said: 'I feel I have to bite my nails or something dreadful may happen', and this in the context was highly suggestive of the act of warding off danger by means of a ritualistic act.

She was a nice girl with reasonable insight into her problem which she understood even more clearly when I explained how trauma during the anal stage can affect people later in life.

These were the suggestions I made to her. First I gave her general 'ego boosting suggestions' to combat her nervousness and lack of confidence, and suggested to her subconscious mind that she would not worry about everyday affairs, nor be frightened when there was no justifiable cause for fear; that the outside world and the empty house would both be acceptable to her, and that she would feel equally relaxed in either.

I then obtained her conscious agreement for me to suggest to her under hypnosis that she would confine her nailbiting to one finger on each hand, for which she selected her forefingers. I made the hypnotic suggestion to her, adding that she was attractive and needed nicely shaped nails to go with her pleasing appearance. I also told her subconscious mind that as her nails grew, she would feel happier and more contented; and added that she would gradually lose the desire to bite even the two permitted fingers. Her obsessive nailbiting ceased after three sessions and at follow-up (three months later) it had not recurred.

This outcome was a fortunate one in some ways. Pollie had bitten her nails for so long the obsessive habit might have been very hard to eradicate; but she was young, bright, easily suggestible and highly motivated, which goes a long way to accounting for the rapid success of the treatment.

Obsessive Trait

The next obsessive patient I will mention, was a twenty-one-year-old girl groom in a local riding school, Annie E. She had a number of problems relating to tension and stress, such as migraine headaches, tense muscles and periodic eating binges, which I think might have had a ritualistic tone to them, for she frequently ate until she vomited — and would then eat more. She loathed being overweight, but continued to eat massive amounts nevertheless.

Her chief complaint, together with lack of confidence and general unhappiness, was an obsession with light switches and gas taps — all of which she had to go back to check several times over although she knew they were safely off.

Annie had had a very strict upbringing, with more severity from her father than from mother with whom she got on well. She had never slept well, and had had recurrent bad dreams of being bombed and hiding in the rubble; she feared violence and aggression of all kinds and definitely took a great deal of unreasonable behaviour from her father who was very unkind to her. Her mother tended to be a person of extremes, and to be very anxious about cleanliness and had, it appeared, been a bit harsh about soiling when Annie was three to four years of age. She had been separated from her mother for several months from the age of one year onwards, since her mother had had to go into hospital. She could never remember feeling happily confident, and wished to overcome her obsessive habits.

My therapy for Annie was to ease her tension and establish confidence by inducing a very relaxed state during hypnosis and then teaching her to do the same at home using autohypnosis. Her obsession with taps and switches gradually faded, as the anxiety levels diminished; she had only had the habit for eighteen months and the feeling that it warded off 'something horrible' for the same length of time.

Her headaches improved and we reduced her weight slightly. She began to feel more confident at work and in social groups, and started to realize that she needed to leave home and assert her own will-power more; also that she would tend to overeat for the element of comfort, all the time she lived at home and encountered her father on a daily basis. Unfortunately Annie was made redundant and had to cease coming for sessions of therapy despite an arrangement to help her financially.

Obsessive Symptoms

Many patients present themselves to hypnotherapists, not as clearcut textbook cases but as a complex mixture of several different forms of disturbance. Marleen K. was one such person, for besides her chief complaint of agoraphobia and her lack of confidence, plus her anxiety attacks when alone at home, she suffered badly from an obsessive desire to start and restart the engine of the car outside. She frequently checked the telephone to see whether it was working and the electric lights to see whether there had been a power cut; but her most troublesome obsession was with having to start and restart the car engine, at all times of the day and night. Her husband had tried leaving the car in the garage or in a nearby field (they were a farming family) but she got so anxious and desperate that he stopped doing this after one or two attempts.

Marleen was thirty-two when she came for treatment. She gave a life story with plenty of evidence in it regarding the development of her phobia, but here I am presenting only those details of her story and the subsequent treatment that pertain to obsessive behaviour. She was happily married but often felt lonely, and was bewildered by her need for ritual and by her fears.

The protective ritual had started after an incident when she was fifteen — the first obsession was with checking the tyres of her bicycle and pumping them up extremely often; later when she started to drive, her obsession centred upon the car rather than on the bicycle. Shortly after her fifteenth birthday, she had been left alone to look after her parents' petrol station in the depths of the country. Her sister called on her and she decided to walk down to the village leaving her sister in charge.

On the way she passed a dirty repulsive-looking tramp and she ran home. Her sister left and when she was alone in the house she saw the tramp coming along towards the house — she felt petrified and ran out into the road to the protection of a woodcutter attending to the hedges — and stayed with him until her parents returned. A couple of years later her uncle of whom she was very fond, died on her birthday — and in the same year her first child was born. After this event, she started to experience panic (anxiety) attacks, and her protection ritual (she herself called it that) became more deeply obsessional and more demanding on her.

Hypnotherapeutic treatment consisted initially of confidence building and ego strengthening; she was regressed to the age of fifteen and revivified the tramp incident, at which she became distressed — but had been strengthened in preparation for this, by the suggestion that it would be something she could handle.

We also went back in time to just after the birth of her first child; her mother in law had been living with her and her husband at the time and had completely taken the child over, causing Marleen much anger which she repressed, and a lot of resentment. She revivified this incident too, again with the protection of ego-boosting to help her handle it, and she released much pent-up anger and grief.

After these two abreactions, the ritualistic behaviour was disposed of, there being no further need of it. Clearly she was predisposed to obsessiveness during her early childhood — but the ritual had been adopted after the terrifying tramp incident, and maintained after her uncle's death and her first child's birth, to fend off from consciousness the anger and resentment and hostility she felt towards her husband's mother.

Her anxiety attacks ceased and so did her phobia of fields and open spaces and crowds, after I had approached this part of her disturbance by means of deep relaxation and lessons in autohypnosis.

Obsessional Person

The following patient is one who stands out among the other obsessional types, because her obsessional pattern was chiefly one involving thought processes rather than ritualistic activity.

Patsy F. came to see me, distressed with thoughts that would not leave her. She was a twenty-eight-year-old housewife who had been married for four years. She wanted to have a baby, but was scared to do so, in case she killed it; she wanted to kill her relations, and her husband whom she loved dearly, and she hated and despised herself because of these thoughts. In addition to the obsession with murder, Patsy was scared of going into town to shop, and would get an anxiety attack when faced with the prospect.

Her husband was a surveyor, and was puzzled but sympathetic about her 'nerves' — he knew nothing about her obsessional thoughts. Both Patsy's parents were dead; nevertheless, she had numerous relatives living in the area. Patsy's father had died when she was twelve, and he had been a strict and puritanical disciplinarian; after his death her mother had started to 'enjoy herself' and one night, when Patsy was just thirteen, she had gone downstairs to get a glass of milk and had seen her mother half naked in the arms of a strange man. She was very shocked.

When Patsy was fourteen her mother went away for a week; and left her in charge of the house with her brother. One night her brother came home drunk, and indecently assaulted her, threatening her next morning that if the relatives found out they would reject her like they were rejecting their mother. Her brother went to live elsewhere a few months later and one year later her mother died; Patsy went to live with an aunt. The aunt made her very unhappy by referring to her mother as a loose woman, and telling Patsy she would go the same way. Patsy left and found a flat of her own where she was far happier.

However, she began to have dreams of a sexual masochistic nature, and nightmares which had legal punishment and prison as a recurring theme. A year or two later she married her boss, who, she said, was 'a charming man, and all a woman could wish for'.

Her first obsessional thoughts occurred shortly after her marriage, when her brother who had returned for a weekend visit and was staying with a cousin, suddenly walked into the kitchen on a surprise visit. Patsy was peeling potatoes at the time and suddenly felt that she wanted to stick the knife into her brother's heart. Her brother left before long and soon went abroad, but Patsy's thoughts continued and grew to embrace all her relations; she started to get panic attacks before visits to relations and before going shopping. This was the state of affairs when she first came for treatment.

Patsy was an excellent hypnotic subject. We started with some ego strengthening and went on to ideomotor signalling, i.e., the use of a forefinger movement to indicate 'yes' or 'no' to a question asked under an hypnotic trance condition; this is often easier for the patient than actually talking under hypnosis. I discovered during the ideomotor sessions, that Patsy was scared to have a child 'in case it grew up like her'; this I interpreted as a subconscious acceptance of guilt.

I regressed her to the scene of assault by her brother, and this caused an abreaction, with tears and cries of distress; she was buffered against too much dis'ress, however, by pre-abreaction suggestions of ability to cope. This released Patsy's guilt, and afterwards we were able to discuss freely her relationship with and attitude towards her mother — her anger and shock were released by abreaction, as was her resentment towards the aunt who had made her miserable during her stay with her.

Patsy finally agreed to confide in her husband about the incident with her brother — her husband was very understanding and she lost her obsessional preoccupation with a wish to murder. This I put down, I am sure correctly, to a desperate desire to preserve the security of her marriage, murdering brother and other relations if and when necessary; and fearing to go to town, because of whom she might meet.

Soon after the cessation of her obsessional thoughts, Patsy stopped having panic attacks, and last time we saw her, she was happily pregnant and looking forward to the birth of her child.

Hypochondriacal Symptoms

Next we have the case of Billy H., a thirty-four-year-old engineer who came on his doctor's advice and was complaining of what he called 'nervous stomach'. He had an eight year history of gastro-intestinal pain and an overactive bowel, as he called it, which in fact meant that he had unexplained bouts of diarrhoea in the morning before leaving for work. All of Billy's symptoms were inexplicable, in fact, at least so far as his doctor and the hospital were concerned, for he had had every test, investigation and X-ray in the book, every single one of which was negative.

Sundry medicines had been prescribed for him to alleviate his complaint — none of which worked — and he had also seen a psychiatrist who had prescribed an antidepressant drug for him, which also failed to help. Billy himself felt, he told me, that there was an organic cause for his ills, and described his symptoms in minute detail, emphasizing all the while that he was a 'difficult case', a fact he really seemed to relish. Besides seeing numerous NHS doctors, he had paid to consult specialists privately and had also done the rounds of the fringe therapies.

None of the forms of 'alternative medicine' had done anything for him either, and he seemed to take a delight in the obstinacy of his symptoms, of which he was obviously proud. Although he assured me that nothing so far prescribed had done him any good, he was currently taking nine different preparations when he came to consult me, from homoeopathic remedies to herbal preparations, plus of course some orthodox pills and potions.

There had been no untoward sex incidents in Billy's early life, and at the time of our meeting he was happily married. He said that he was a placid sort of fellow who did not like rows or signs of aggression. He had had a strict upbringing by Plymouth Brethren parents, and had always been submissive to them, never disobedient or recalcitrant. He trained as an engineer because that was what his father had wanted him to do, and was happy in his present job, but between the ages of twenty-two and thirty years he had worked for a firm he detested.

He had always worked hard and very conscientiously, but had been exploited by his boss, an unpleasant and jealous man who had passed over Billy's name when promotion was in the offing. His boss actually told him one day that 'he would never get anywhere in life'. He stuck to the job for eight years until his wife persuaded him to change. He was scared to do so at first, because he was very security-conscious and careful about earning and saving money, but finally took the bull by the horns. The change of job had not been easy but Billy was very happy in his present employment; unfortunately, though, he still had his complaints, which had started shortly after his boss had told him he would always be a failure.

I suggested to him during the course of our discussion, that he had repressed hostility still, towards his former employer, and a fear of authority stemming from childhood, the two concurrent feelings producing a conflict which could account for his present symptoms, partly as an understandable, silent protest, and partly as a subconscious method of ego compensation; I meant by this, that he had a subconscious need to assert himself as a result of unjust treatment and unrecognized ability over the years, for which his present contentment in his job only partially compensated. And because, as a true hypochondriac and anal type of personality, he almost totally lacked aggression, the part of him that needed to express his anger had to find an outlet that his mentality could find acceptable. Hence the symptoms.

It is very unlikely that a hypnotherapist would tell any patient that he was a hypochondriac! To the therapist the term is not an accusation but the name of a diagnosis for a condition requiring treatment, but so many of the common diagnostic terms — hypochondriac, schizoid, hysteric, paranoid — have personally insulting connotations, or at the very least, the ability to make the patient unhappy and worried and therefore worse than he was to start off with. So I was very careful how I explained Billy's symptoms when I was talking to him, picking up any shreds of evidence where I could from his history of disturbance during his anal phase of development.

It appeared that with his parents, cleanliness was next to godliness, and neither parent had been able to tolerate the fact that Billy was not 'clean' almost from birth! There had been multiple scoldings, spankings and punishments from about the age of one year to the age of seven, at which age he had still soiled himself from time to time. Mercifully a year at a boarding school where he was accepted and very happy, intervened, and he was cured of the soiling. Not, however, of course, of the conflicts that had arisen during those years due to the excessive discipline and love withdrawal.

My treatment was to strengthen Billy's ego, and to regress him to an early age in childhood so that he could revivify some of the disciplinary incidents. He abreacted at this stage with a lot of emotion released, as also happened when we went back to the stage in his career when his boss told him that he was and always would be a failure. As I had suspected, he had bottled up a great deal of understandable resentment at these words, coming from someone he felt he ought to respect and for whom he had done his more than adequate best. I also made the suggestion that aggression under certain circumstances could be a good thing and that he would be better able to stand up for himself in the future.

We eased his habitual tension by relaxation sessions and I suggested to him, while in a medium to deep trance, that now he had released pent-up emotion and had a great deal more insight into his problem, his mind no longer needed the symptoms it was producing and that they could therefore leave him. Moreover, that the pride he had felt in his symptoms because they made him feel important and special, would be converted into pride in his new ability to deal with people and the world about him. I suggested to him a feeling of warmth creeping over the usually painful area of his abdomen, and taught him for good measure to recreate the same sensation at home under autohypnosis.

His bowel function returned to normal and he had one regular motion daily, instead of three or four trips to the lavatory before leaving for work each day. Billy grew more confident and relaxed and his pain symptoms diminished considerably. Last time I saw him for follow-up, the bouts of pain had grown less and less frequent, and he was confident that they would soon disappear altogether.

Many hypnotherapists find that hypochondriac patients are not a particularly easy group of patients to treat. But they can often be persuaded to relinquish their symptoms if there is an incident within their childhood or even their later history which can account for their need for those symptoms. For, together with increased insight and awareness, plus of course abreaction of the incident(s) where indicated, comes the ability to 'leave go' of ailments as the need for them ceases.

Sometimes, though, no amount of probing succeeds in bringing to light any apparent cause for such a need and the problem is a great one for the therapist and the patient alike. Suggestions can be made that the symptoms will disappear and be replaced by 'a warm glow' etc. — which the patient can be taught to generate. This is successful in a number of hypochondriacs.

8. Genital Conflicts

The third stage of psychological development initially postulated by Freud, is the 'genital' phase, which takes over from the anal phase at around the age of three years. Also known as the 'phallic-oedipal' period, it is characterized by the child's increasing awareness of his or her own genital organs, accompanied by curiosity and anxiety with respect to sexual differences. It is a period of time when the youngster may develop passionate feelings for the parent of the opposite sex, with correspondingly aggressive feelings towards any individual who appears to threaten or rival the situation.

It is helpful for parents to be aware of this likely chain of events, for young mothers often become very distressed and sometimes angry, at the puzzling attitude adopted by a usually very affectionate four-year-old daughter in which she fights against Mother's wishes all the time and has eyes only for Daddy. Fathers, too, can become puzzled and upset at their young son's antagonistic feelings towards them, for no reason that is apparent — coupled with a sudden intense devotion to Mummy and the constant desire to please her.

This phase is followed by 'latency', which is a spell of disinterest in sexuality, during which the child's attention is far more engrossed with getting on with his peer group, learning processes at school, and outside activities involving hobbies and sports. The latent period ends as puberty commences due to hormone production, and the genital phase proper begins.

Harm to the developing and maturing psyche, results from early but genuine sexual feelings being transformed into feelings of guilt. There are many ways in which this can come about, and the damage that results from such a transformation expresses itself later in life, in one of two ways. The first of these is hysteria, and the second is anxiety neurosis (the anxiety state). There are innumerable ways in which hysteria can make itself manifest, as we shall see. And anxiety states can cause genuine physical disease, phobias, great and incapacitating fears and sexual disorders such as impotence and frigidity.

What are the causes for this unhealthy way of developing? In theory, a more sexually liberated society such as we live in today, should bring about fewer neuroses due to transformation of true sexual feeling into guilt, than was the case up to, say, the middle sixties, when a broader view and more relaxed attitude to sexual behaviour was beginning to take a firm root. Whether this will be proven by time, we have yet to see, but regardless of society's attitude to adult sex, it still offends parents to see small children fingering their genital organs during the 'phallic-oedipal' years — and in fact are just as likely to scold or smack the child for so doing, if it happens at home as they are if it occurs in a public place.

It is true that the habit is regarded as 'antisocial' and many older people dislike watching a toddler preoccupied in touching and playing with his or another child's penis, or exploring below skirt level in the case of little girls. The best method, to me, seems to be to explain to the child as soon as it can understand you, in very simple terms, that it is better not to play games, touch, rub oneself in front of other people, and that the privacy of his/her bedroom is the right place for such activities if they feel they have to follow them. At the same time, gently stressing that you are not 'angry', and that they are not 'dirty', 'naughty' or 'unlovable' just because they are curious.

Similarly when small children asks questions about where babies come from, why Johnny is shaped differently from his sister, tell one another dirty jokes etc. — it can make all the difference to their healthy development, to be taken seriously and answered in a manner they understand, rather than scolded into a condition of enforced secrecy and guilt.

Hysteria

In many ways, it would be a good thing if a new term could be coined for the psychological condition known to psychiatrists and psychologists as hysteria. By it, a doctor or therapist is referring to a personality type, and the full diagnostic term is: 'hysterical personality'. But nowadays patients quite rightly demand to know exactly what is wrong with them or their sick relation, and when told that the diagnosis is one of hysteria, they tend to look askance.

This is due to the fact that the word is still associated, in the minds of many of us, with an attack similar to the Victorian vapours but characterized in particular by screaming, laughing, weeping and flinging oneself about all over the place. When people describe something as 'hysterical' they generally mean that it is productive of uncontrollable laughter; and when they claim to have become practically hysterical in a given situation, they are referring to having been on the verge of a panic attack, with the accompanying feelings of unpleasant excitement and the tendency to shout, cry or laugh as a way of unburdening mounting tension.

The fullblown attack of 'hysteria' as described above, is only one possible manifestation of a complex and many faceted complaint, and is now known as 'classical hysteria', or 'la grande hysterie'. The illness itself, or abnormally developed personality, is in fact a way of reacting to difficulties encountered by the individual — and appears as often in men as it does in women. In essence it consists of producing by *unconscious means* an alarming physical or mental state in oneself, with the aim of manipulating people and/or events which have not been controlled by other means.

On the surface this seems to be a contradiction in terms. How can anybody employ a means of achieving their own ends, in the face of opposing people or events, without it being malingering and fraudulent? The answer is that what looks like unscrupulous behaviour to a normal person with ordinary insight, is entirely unconscious so far as the true hysteric is concerned, as he/she has no insight whatever, and no idea at all that he possesses ulterior motives. Such a person is almost always of a very low cultural background and the illness of hysteria is believed never to be found among people who are well developed mentally, educationally and emotionally.

The unconscious intentions of a hysterical person, are to coerce by means of terrifying or shocking, so that the children, parents, boss or best friend give in to their demands. It is a hallmark of hysteria, that if their unconscious demands are met with, fresh and further symptoms follow so that more can be gained for the individual; whereas ignoring the condition results in its disappearing, at least temporarily.

Here are some of the reasons for the production of hysteria: (1) an inadequate individual may resent the lack of attention he receives, and compel attention from others by producing a dramatic illness; (2) as a means of getting people to comply with his/her wishes, as mentioned above; (3) as a desperate though unconscious attempt to avoid responsibility, so that the 'symptoms' or 'illness' can be blamed for poor performance and not the individual him/herself. Hysterical people like always to be provided with a scapegoat they can blame for their own failings and shortcomings; symptoms are used when there is no preferable alternative. And (4), hysterical symptoms may be used to attract the sympathy of someone upon whom the individual depends for a supply of effort and vitality — this is reminiscent of the activity of the vampire of mythology, and in fact is known by psychologists as 'vampirism'.

Hysteria generally produces florid physical symptoms, and while these may be most alarming to friends and relations, a doctor will generally smell a rat because the average hysteric has to depend upon his/her own knowledge of actual clinical symptomatology as stored in his/her subconscious mind. As the genuine hysteric is not a malingerer, there is no question of his going to the library and looking up medical textbooks in order to produce a convincing array of signs and symptoms. He is unlikely to produce a convincing picture of a given disease, in fact, unless he has for some reason had cause to study anatomy or disease processes in the past. But, whether apparently genuine illness or transparent symptoms are in evidence, the state is known as 'conversion-hysteria' because a trouble that really exists in the mind of the person is 'converted' into physical signs.

A wide range of such illnesses exist, including asthma; migraine; paralysis; loss of the power of speech, hearing, smell etc.; and though the knowledge used to produce them may be memory-stored subconsciously or present in the conscious mind, the *process* by which it is utilized in the production of appropriate symptoms is in itself unconscious. When the conversion has been successful, however, hysterics do consciously trade upon their skill and embellish the illness with all types of lurid details.

When ignored, the 'symptoms' tend to disappear. But although the hysteric may well then forget all about his illness and get on with life, bearing no particular grudge because he has been seen through — he is just as likely to try again when the circumstance seems right for him to do so.

Another feature common to hysterical conversion illnesses, is the extreme appropriateness of the adopted complaint to the requirements of the hysterical person. A woman encouraged to take her driving test before she feels ready for it — and to whom it is a major and very significant event — may well dread the occasion so much that the morning of the test produces real and unpleasant symptoms of an asthma attack — under which conditions she clearly couldn't drive anywhere. A person entertaining a secret dread of speechmaking who is invited to speak at an event it is impossible not to attend, may well 'convert' his mental trouble into an attack of laryngitis in which he genuinely cannot raise his voice above a whisper.

Medical treatment has a notable effect upon hysterical illnesses — it is notable for its total lack of success! While the patient may appear anxious to receive treatment, as this convinces those around him that he is genuinely ill, he has no desire at all to have the ailment leave him and has two aims in mind only — the first is the 'primary gain', which consists of the successful manipulation of people and events, and the second is that of 'secondary gain', consisting of the extra care, consideration and sympathy he or she attracts on account of receiving professional treatment for the illness. So no hysteric is really at all concerned with his or her apparently serious illness, and has no wish at all to recover.

Not all psychosomatic illness is produced by hysteria — far from it. As we shall see from our account of anxiety neurosis, real diagnosable physical disease processes can be produced in the body as a direct result of this particular mental syndrome, and the duodenal ulcer, gastritis, muscular pain etc. engendered by the anxiety are as real and demonstrable as they would be if they were to arise from entirely different causes. But no real evidence of disease can be found in a hysteric because, of course, he is perfectly well apart from mentally.

Mention should be made, in passing, of hysterical dissociation, although it is not a common condition compared with the others discussed. It is present in cases of people with a 'split personality', a phrase often erroneously used with reference to schizophrenics. An excellent example of hysterical dissociation, is the fictional character(s) Doctor Jekyll and Mr Hyde — one benevolent, the other psychopathic, and neither aware of the existence of the other. The characteristic feature of this curious condition is the existence of two or more personalities all quite different from one another, and slipped into by the individual more or less at random without his or her conscious knowledge that anything is amiss.

Hence a man may be a truck-driver one minute, a film star celebrity a bit later on, and (so he thinks) a landscape gardener the next day. While living within one role, he is absolutely unaware that the rest exist, and he plays that part perfectly and unto the manner born until he is precipitated into the next role.

The simplest form of this complaint is sleep-walking or somnambulism, in which there is no breakdown into other characters but words are spoken and actions performed during sleep, of which the person has not the faintest recollection on waking. This is a lot commoner than true hysterical dissociation.

Would you know a hysterical person if you met one? A hysteric remains a hysteric even though he may not be showing any overt symptoms, and this type of personality has some characteristics that can enable a doctor or specialist to recognize him in the absence of actual hysterical symptoms.

Typically a man or woman with a hysterical make-up, is an extroverted, materialistic sort of person who attaches enormous value to money and possessions and yet lacks intellectual or spiritual depths, and any degree of intuitive power or insight. He is childlike and simple, highly suggestible and highly dramatic in the way he coverts the limelight and is never out of it if he can avoid it. He can make extravagant gèstures meant to express deep attachment and emotional depths, but this is just another pose, for such a person is incapable of real attachment and depths of feeling, and is in fact a pauper in the emotional sense, with nothing to offer and no real ability to keep and cherish that which is offered to him.

The hysterical person sets an enormous amount of store on admiration. Not having the capacity for a deep two-way relationship, he actually prefers frank admiration to love, or at least if he receives love from a partner then the element of it he most appreciates is that of overt admiration. Because he lacks insight into his own personality, he does not for a moment suppose that anyone will notice the deep well of materialistic values and emotional poverty behind his striking façade of extroversion and role playing.

When life is suiting him, the hysteric can be good company, indeed the 'life and soul of the party', as he loves an audience, the physical pleasures of good food, wine and entertainment, and the change and stimulation of social gatherings. When facing a reversal of fortune however, his cheery manner breaks down and his shallow and inept self is revealed. Never — ever — being in the wrong, the hysteric will always be able to drum up a scapegoat, for loss of face to him, or having to admit to an error of judgement, are more terrible prospects than anything else he can envisage. If faced with a situation in which no scapegoat is apparent then his subconscious mind will produce symptoms to blame, and to cajole people with. A frothy exterior hides an almost total vacuum within.

The Anxiety State

This is a common condition and a very unpleasant one. Its chief and most obvious characteristic is the feeling of anxiety experienced by the individual, for which no reason is apparent. Because the anxious person is unconscious of any reason for his anxiety, the anxiety itself is called 'unconscious'. This is an abnormal state, as it cannot be related to anything of which the person is aware. Worry, on the other hand, while often as unpleasant, is normal as the worrying person can at once tell you what it is that is concerning him.

Worry and anxiety are different in another way. A person worried by something, will take appropriate action to deal with the problem; the anxious person can do no such thing as he or she knows of no reason causing the feeling of which he is complaining. So instead of anxiety prompting recourse to alleviating action, it gives rise instead to symptoms and the anxiety reaction.

An anxiety attack brings on certain bodily symptoms which terrify the anxious person, in contrast to the symptoms of a hysteric, about which he is happily unconcerned. The anxiety symptoms are similar to those provoked by a 'normal' situation in which fear would be appropriate, such as being chased by an Alsatian, or seeing a ghost. The person knows of nothing causing the symptoms he experiences, and is very frightened by his dry mouth, rapidly beating heart, a feeling of suffocation, rigidity of the muscles and perhaps cold perspiration if the attack is a severe one. Such an attack is terrible to experience and can be frightening to observe. The anxious person is usually unable to speak for a while and can only manage afterwards to do so with great difficulty.

He experiences great suffering of the body and the mind (introversion), whereas the hysteric by contrast suffers no discomfort himself but tries to extort sympathy from his audience. The unpleasant mental activity associated with an anxiety attack, is neither true thought nor identifiable feeling; it is an absence of usual adult mental activity, which in itself is terrifying, and has most nearly been described as the mental interpretation of a bodily state. This is the condition Freud called 'free floating anxiety', because it is free from any logical explanation and 'floats' before the mind of the person without attaching itself to an object, person or circumstance.

Once an anxiety attack has occurred for the first time, it will recur because of the impression it makes on the mind and the fact that it leaves memory traces and a pattern that is likely to be repeated. The attack is the outward sign that in the deep recesses of the unconscious, internal conflict is occurring, and continues to occur despite the occasional release of tension afforded by the attack.

The result of this inner conflict is the feeling of anxiety and unease that the anxiety victim has to face every day of his life. The energy builds up and affects his autonomic nervous system and glands and produces the bodily state that is ready to cope with a 'fight or flight' state, except the person cannot discharge the energy by actually fighting or fleeing for he is unaware of the basic cause. This is the reason for the perpetual feelings of impending disaster such people experience — and the inner tension continues to mount until it is again discharged in an anxiety attack.

The secret to interpreting the anxiety attack lies in the close parallel between it and the sexual act. If this sounds odd — think how in the normal act, excitement increases in intensity to the accompaniment of pleasurable bodily sensations, which further raise the excitement level — until the generated energy reaches its height and spills over in the orgasm, the climax of the act. An anxiety attack has mounting tension, another form of energy; (unpleasant) physical symptoms are produced, and these play on the mental state, increasing the mounting tension, until the energy spills over and is discharged in an anxiety attack. The significance of this close parallel, is that it indicates the true nature of the anxiety attack: it is a distorted way of releasing sexual energy, which cannot be channelled in the normal way because this outlet has been denied to it.

This means that both normal sexuality and the anxiety attack are expressions of the sexual instinct. They are also both related to the other primitive instinct of self-preservation, for the part of the nervous system designed to cope with fight or flight mechanisms when the individual is faced by physical threat, i.e., when self-preservation is threatened, is the same part as the one that deals with anxiety attacks. In an anxiety attack, then, normal sexual energy is converted into the distorted reactions of fear, discomfort and panic. The result is that in such a person, anxiety will inevitably be bound up with sexual activity and expression.

Our minds deal with the constant burden of anxiety by developing symptoms of one kind or another to which the 'free floating anxiety' can be related. It is an intolerable state of affairs to have ever-mounting tension, which can be related to no identifiable cause, and so the mind produces something to represent, i.e., symbolize, the actual unknown reason for the attacks.

The way chosen in a particular individual, is determined by the personality type and the particular symbolism with which his subconscious mind is used to dealing. There are three possibilities:

1. In the form of a bodily symptom
Bodily symptoms are an inseparable part of a true anxiety attack. Any one body system may be unconsciously elected there and then at the time of the first attack, to develop symptoms to which the anxiety can consciously be attached. If supposing the person had had a car accident when a child, and had had recurrent headaches on and off since that time — this potentially weak area might be singled out and further symptoms engendered with the head becoming the focal point for symbolic symptoms to develop.

In doing this, unbearable anxiety has been dealt with by providing a 'reason' for the unattached anxiety; such symptoms are generally treated with medicines and even surgery, but the problem standing in the way of success, is that medication can only succeed in controlling the symptom, it cannot reach the underlying cause of the trouble.

2. Phobias
Intellectually developed 'anxiety types' of people tend to develop phobias, which are a clever attempt at reaching a solution to the

problem of free floating anxiety by substituting the known (a fear that develops and attaches itself to an object in the external environment) for the unknown. It is the mental parallel of the attempt to substitute bodily symptoms for the unknown cause.

When formless anxiety is attached to 'something' external to the person it is easier to tolerate and allows the individual to take appropriate action, i.e., avoidance of the thing to which the phobia has developed, be it closed spaces, crowds, open spaces, mice, spiders or cats. And all the time that the object arousing phobic symptoms is avoided, the person is free from anxiety.

The problem with the phobic solution, is that the process of symbolism soon extends itself into a wider class, and therefore is harder to avoid. For instance, fear of enclosed spaces will probably extend from a dislike of entering the cupboard under the stairs to fear of going inside the house at all.

3. Concern for others

The third way in which unconscious anxiety is dealt with, is by externalization and identification. The free floating anxiety is identified with the real problems and worries of other people, about which the afflicted person worries a great deal. Certainly the process is entirely unconscious, but this does not obviate the worry, misery and concern he feels on the behalf of others. This is the best of the three solutions as although the troubles of other people only symbolize the person's own — at least satisfaction can be gained by helping them and watching their problems disappear, thus symbolically removing the cause of the anxiety personally felt.

We will now look at some case histories and problems of people who have suffered from hysteria and from anxiety neurosis.

9. Case Histories of Genital Types

In an ordinary day-to-day hypnotherapy practice in this country the average hypnotherapist does not come across a great deal of hysteria among the patients he treats. There are probably two reasons for this. First, there are far greater numbers of ordinary, uncomplicated, reasonably well-balanced people who wish quite simply to lose weight, give up smoking, cease to bite their nails or receive some counselling/confidence boosting, than there are individuals who exhibit hysterical conversion symptoms in a subconscious attempt to control their environment. And second, as we noted in the last chapter, the last person to be worried by the symptoms of hysterical conversion syndrome is the hysteric himself.

He is *not* concerned about whether he will soon recover, and is not anxiously seeking out new forms of therapy, as perhaps might the hypochondriac or the 'anxiety state' patient who is worried to death by his symptoms. The hysteric is not at all anxious to be cured of his paralysis, his loss of speech or his asthma attacks; they serve far too useful a purpose to be dismissed from his life.

Here are two instances among our records of hysterical patients who *have* come for treatment:

Hysteria (1)

Paul J. was a twenty-three-year-old naval officer who had seen active service in the Falklands. The symptom of which he was complaining was an uncontrollable muscular action in his left leg which would come on when he was sitting or lying down, and sometimes when he was standing still. It consisted of an involuntary sideways kicking motion, which looked and felt ridiculous to his conscious mind and was sufficient to threaten seriously his chance of remaining in the navy. He had had the problem for about a year when I first saw him, and it had troubled him since shortly after his ship had sunk.

During a hypnotic trance Paul remembered the causative event which was hazy to the memory of his conscious mind. During the sea attack in which his ship had been destroyed, he had been on deck and had seen several of his colleagues blown to pieces in front of him. He himself had been knocked over by the blast and severely bruised, and at one point in time, as flames from a blazing tarpaulin were threatening to engulf him, he had kicked out defiantly with his left leg, in a valiant attempt to ward off the flames.

He had failed in his attempt and had been burned on the feet and lower legs before fainting from shock. When he came to, he had been saved from the fire on deck and the sinking ship by his superior officer. He had recovered from the first and second degree burns, but at the time of his rehabilitation back in England, the strange kicking motion had started.

The kicking motion was exactly that which would have been required to save him from the approaching fire. He had been emotionally very shocked by the sight of his colleagues being killed and the fear of apparently approaching death by fire — and the muscular kicking action remained with him as a means of getting him away from the scene of the trauma and as a result of stored up anger at the death around him and the hopelessness of the situation. Although this was a form of hysterical conversion to suit the immediate need, Paul was not a characteristic full-blown hysterical personality, and once the purpose had been served, he was genuinely anxious to return to full service.

I aided him to abreact, by revivifying the incident and releasing all the pent-up fear, anger and desperation that the original situation had engendered. During abreaction, as he lay on the couch in a hypnotic trance and relived the terror of the sea battle, he cried, screamed, shouted, swore and kicked about with both legs as the 'flames' approached — especially with his left leg.

After I brought him out of hypnotic trance I asked him to report back to me in one week. He did so, and had only been troubled by one brief 'kicking' session.

I implanted the post-hypnotic suggestion, that neither fatigue nor tension would be capable of causing a relapse in the future, as the more stressful his immediate circumstances the more easily he would be able to cope and the more capable he would know himself to be. This put an end to the trouble and there was no recurrence of the involuntary kicking movement.

Hysteria (2)

The second case of hysteria I will give an account of was an interesting one of hysterical blindness. This type of hysterical conversion is a reaction to unbearable circumstances which stimulate the inner conflicts we know already exist within hysterics to enable them to undergo hysterical conversion phenomena in the first place.

Joan S. was blind, and had been so for five years following a motor accident in which her husband and two children had been killed in the car in which the four of them were travelling. The motorway accident had involved a terrible scene with a jack-knifing truck, and only Joan had been spared — after the appalling experience of witnessing the death by crushing of her family, only a few feet away.

She had, of course, been taken to hospital and treated for severe shock — only to discover to her horror three days later that she could not see properly. She had never had any trouble with her sight, and went to an ophthalmic specialist who could find nothing organically wrong with her eyes. Her pupils reacted to light with pupillary contraction, and even she admitted that she experienced remissions and exacerbations which occurred spontaneously for no apparent cause.

Her case history revealed the right background for a possible hysterical reaction — the death of both parents when she was only four — again in a car accident — and her subsequent education until the age of eighteen in a convent, where the attitude to exploratory sex and early physical curiosity, was that 'it was all works of the Devil', and her subsequent sexual education had consisted of guilty searchings in dictionaries and the occasional 'banned' book.

There was no doubt, though, that the present blindness was caused by the dreadful scene to which she had been a horrified witness. So, hard though it was on Joan, I took her back under hypnotic trance to the motorway scene and got her to rewitness the scene as it really was. She became as one might expect, extremely upset — but I had told her beforehand under hypnosis that she would be able to face up to and cope with any incident she came across in her memory, however painful.

When she 'reached' the scene of the disaster I exhorted her to look and see what was happening, instead of hiding her eyes in her hands as she had apparently done at the time. It was very hard for her to do so, even under hypnotic suggestion, but she accepted my suggestions and did as I wished her to. She portrayed as she did so, her immense feeling of helplessness at the scene of the disaster, and the fact that she had been so shocked she had simply stood stock still in the road, instead of running to help the injured.

After the abreaction was well and truly over and — I felt — utilized in full, I suggested to her that her sight would return just as it had been before the accident had occurred. Not all cases of hysterical conversion respond immediately to one abreaction session, but Joan did so, and her hysterical blindness left her.

Anxiety State (1)

Gaye P. provides me with a case to relate that is practically a 'textbook' account of an anxiety state, how it comes to develop, the bodily symptoms such a condition can produce, and what can be done about the situation, mentally and with respect to the organic symptoms.

Gaye came to see me on the advice of her doctor, who had been investigating her symptoms of stomach pain, nausea, waterbrash and heartburn. As he supposed, she was suffering from a peptic (duodenal) ulcer, and this was confirmed by a barium meal at the hospital, as well as gastroscopy (viewing the interior of the stomach with a lighted tube and lens, while the patient is under mild sedation), as sometimes Gaye's symptoms were very severe and the hospital surgeon wished to eliminate a possible gastric ulcer as well.

Fortunately her stomach lining was normal; but the problem remained of her lack of a satisfactory response to diet, antacids, other peptic ulcer drugs and ceasing to smoke. She would recover for a time, and then the symptoms would start all over again.

I learned from taking a case history from her, that she was a twenty-nine-year-old mother of two, divorced three years previously since her husband had left her for another woman, and that she had always 'been an anxious type of person'. According to Gaye's mother, when she questioned her about previous stomach trouble, Gaye had been a difficult feeder as a baby and small child, and had had a propensity for developing 'tummy trouble'. Later, she often felt sick and had diarrhoea before examinations, and worry about anything gave her heartburn long before she developed a full blown picture of peptic ulceration.

With respect to her childhood, I felt the fact that her parents were 'very strict', that she had not learned about reproduction until the age of twelve because her mother wouldn't discuss the subject, and the terrible row that had ensued at home when she had wanted to go out on her first date at the age of sixteen could safely be tied up with what I was sure was repressed anxiety about sex. She had not enjoyed love-making with her husband, who had been her first lover — and she had not had an affair since. It is always more satisfactory when a hypnotherapist can see clear support for the probable diagnosis in the patient's early life — as we saw in the last chapter, anxiety states arise due to the mis-channelling of sexual energy into the parallel but abnormal anxiety attack; but cases are not always as clear cut as Gaye's was.

She also told me of attacks of 'feeling awful' when her normally high levels of anxiety and uneasy feelings 'suddenly seemed to rush at her, and overwhelm her'; her heart would hammer away, her pulse race, her mouth go dry and sticky, and her muscles would tense themselves as though she expected the sky to fall on her! This was a clear description of a classical anxiety attack, and it was after she had had three or four of those (which were incidentally always followed by stomach pain) that symptoms of peptic ulceration had started to develop.

I asked her what sort of situations tended to bring on attacks of peptic ulcer pain, and she told me that typically they occurred at weekends when her eldest daughter Sue, aged eleven, went out with her friends to the local ice rink, and sometimes on to a party with other friends from school. She was scared Sue would meet a boy 'and that he would do something nasty to her'. She had tried to avoid being like her mother, and had discussed sex with both daughters, and was as liberal with them as she could bring herself to be — but the very thought that Sue, who was attractive and mature for her age, would be intimate with a boy, brought on the most awful ulcer attacks every time.

This was my campaign of therapy for Gaye. We discussed at length, the actual likelihood of her worst fears being realized; she even brought Sue along to see me and we had a chat, as a result of which I told Gaye that I thought her fears were quite unfounded. But, I pointed out, such things do happen, and it was better that she overcame her fears and tensions about the matter or it could have a bad effect on the girl. We went on to discuss sex and the sex act at length, and I was able to gauge the depths of her distaste and fear of love-making. She had never experienced orgasm, and I suggested some appropriate reading material for her, which placed sex in a realistic light, and explained about orgasms and the absence of them; how sex can be beautiful, joyous and highly pleasurable or just the opposite; and how to encourage orgasms to occur, either in conjunction with a partner or alone.

Then we had some sessions of hypnotic trance, and she proved to be a suggestible subject once she had learned to relax. In fact, relaxation was what I was aiming at getting Gaye to experience, for tension was one of her worst problems; and I suggested to her when she was in a medium depth trance, that she would find, when faced in the future with tension-generating circumstances, that taking slow, deep breaths while saying to herself the words: 'Calmness . . . peace . . . and tranquillity' would take away her anxiety symptoms. I had already got her used to experiencing total relaxation in association with these words, while under hypnosis, and my idea was to plant a post-hypnotic suggestion that she would be able to recreate the relaxed feeling whenever the need arose.

She carried out all that I asked her to do, and there were twelve hypnotic relaxation sessions in all. By this time she was able to tell me that she had had no recurrence of ulcer pain or other symptoms for six weeks, and that she could — and did — utilize the self-induced relaxation technique whenever it was needed. She was also a lot less uptight with her daughters, and not mentally or physically disturbed by Sue's going out. We had two follow up sessions at three-monthly intervals, and the very great improvement had been maintained.

Anxiety State (2)
Bronchial asthma is widely acknowledged to have a strong psychogenic aspect to it, and many workers have found that some cases of asthma are purely psychogenic in origin, with no evidence for allergy as a causative factor anywhere to be found. A personality type has been described as being a common but by

no means invariable finding in such patients; this is highly suggestive of conflicts stemming from the phallic-oedipal or genital proper phases of psychological development, because characteristically the patients repress all their deeper emotions for fear of endangering close relationships, and they frequently are very insecure within the context of sexual activity and sexual partnerships, due to mental conflict about sexuality generally.

Michael Z., a forty-four-year-old builder and decorator, came to see me on the advice of a friend. He owned his own business and was clearly wanting to make a success of it; but frequent asthma attacks were posing a serious threat to this. He had been given every conceivable sensitivity test at the hospital, but no type of allergy could be found. In addition, his own doctor told him that the trouble was probably due to the intense anxiety to which he had always been prey.

Michael told me of typical anxiety attacks which occurred every so often, and also that the asthma attacks themselves had begun when he was just starting puberty. He worried about sex, and did not take a girl out until he was seventeen; his parents had not been overstrict, but one particular master at his school had discovered Michael and two other boys showing their penises to one another in the school lavatory when Michael was seven, and had thrashed all three of them, warning them that they would go to hell if they died and that they were in states of mortal sin (the school was part-monastery).

Michael had not dared to tell his parents, but as soon as he started to get erections and wet dreams, and realize that he was becoming sexually mature, his asthma attacks had started. Even now, he feared the sexual act, and agreed that this was largely why he had never married. He admired one particular lady friend, however, but whenever he even contemplated asking her out for a drink, he would start to wheeze. He felt a sense of doom (free floating anxiety) every day, and although the anxiety attacks had been more or less replaced by the attacks of asthma, nevertheless he still had the occasional one.

We discussed sex at length, and I suggested under hypnosis that the injury inflicted by the master, would cease to have any effect; instead he would start to develop an attraction towards sexual activity, as the fear of the act itself gradually left him. Once Michael realized the significance of the master's irrational and cruel words at an impressionable age, he was more able to understand why his body and mind reacted as they did.

Also, under hypnosis, I gave him regular relaxation, and taught him autohypnosis. Under relaxed, pre-trance conditions I asked him what symbolized peace, beauty and tranquillity for him, and he said candlelight. During the next trance, I got him to visualize a candle flame, and to experience deep peace when so doing, together with the knowledge that his bronchial tubes were also utterly relaxed and that his breathing was easy and unhampered. And I told him that whenever he looked at a candle flame in the future, he would go into a similarly deep state of hypnosis, just by gazing at it and counting backwards from ten to one. When fully relaxed, he would tell himself that his chest was clear of tightness — and would remain so.

I stressed that when he practised this technique at home, he would be able to handle any emergency that might arise for this would automatically bring him out of trance; and that he could bring himself out anyway, when he wished to do so, by counting from one to five. He should do this regularly, and then when faced with a threatening situation on another occasion, simply picturing a candle flame would induce relaxation both of himself and of his air tubes. Michael did as I suggested and found home autohypnosis sessions a great help.

He had one or two further asthma attacks over the next few weeks, and then his ability to cope took over and he was able to control his reactions. Discussion about his earlier life had dispelled much of his conscious tension and tendency to worry about sex, and the relaxation helped to overcome both the anxiety attacks and the asthmatic response. He eventually overcame his fear of sex sufficiently to ask out the girl he was attracted to, and after a year, they married. He has had no further attacks.

Phobic State

In this case we take a look at a typically phobic condition which responded to a hypnotic technique known as systematic desensitization. Phobias are fairly common occurrences and form quite a large portion of the average hypnotherapist's work. Usual ones which we encounter, are claustrophobia (a fear of enclosed spaces); agoraphobia (a fear of seeing many people at once, often amounting to a fear of open spaces); a phobia of spiders; a phobia of the dark; and a phobic fear of cats, dogs (less common), insects other than spiders, and innumerable other objects which the symbology of the patient has endowed with a phobic significance. Frequently, a phobic fear of a particular object or situation can be traced back to an incident in the patient's life in which the feared thing played a major and predominantly terrifying part. But those who adhere to Freudian theory maintain that there is always a part of the individual's development during the genital phase, which has predisposed to phobic fear development in later life. Sometimes, the therapist can identify the object or occurrence, and sometimes this is not possible — but the fact remains that the production of a case of phobia is possible only when trauma has occurred during the genital phase of psychological development, and at least some evidence of this can usually be found in the individual's life history.

Henry O. had a phobia of earthworms. This is not a particularly common phobia, and you might suppose that, since he lived in the City of London, it was a phobia that did not occasion him much discomfort. This was not actually the case, however, as his story will reveal.

Henry lived in London, it is true, but his parents lived in the heart of the Cotswolds, and he returned there as often as he could. He came to consult me because of a very upsetting incident that had occurred during a weekend back home with his family, and there was no way in which I could possibly have dismissed his fears by merely pointing out that he would, after all, encounter earthworms only very infrequently.

Henry O. was a bit of a 'Hurrah Henry' type — but very sincere for all that, and fairly bright, at least as far as the computer firm for which he worked was concerned. He was however, shy of the opposite sex, and had considered it quite a major personal achievement when he had managed to date on three successive weekends the local Huntmaster's daughter, with whom he had been to school, but of whom he had an almost reverential fear of offending. The weekend before he came to see me he had been for a spring walk with the girl through some local woodland, and was just plucking up the necessary courage to propose, when he had been stricken with what, to Henry, practically amounted to a fit.

'We were walking along the path between the beeches,' he told me. 'I had my arm around Isabelle's waist and was just about to pop the important question, when I looked down and spotted this damned earthworm! It had been raining, and the worm was slithering across the path, to get out of our way, I suppose. I only know, that when I saw it, I experienced the most awful panic attack and felt sick, and had to turn away. Isabelle immediately noticed that something was wrong and led me back to the Landrover; but I felt a terrible fool, and feeling dependent instead of weak is not encouraging when one is trying to ask a girl to marry one!'

I took his point; in Henry's world, that admittedly so many of us inhabit, men were supposed to be the strong members of the family, and capable of defending their wives and children; certainly not individuals who felt mortally ill at the sight of a mere worm.

I was most intrigued by Henry's story, as well as anxious to help him, and further questioning sessions revealed the following information. When he was nine years old, he had been for a walk with his two older boy cousins, and they had relieved themselves in a brook over which their walk took them. He had noticed the size of their penises (they were twelve and thirteen respectively) and had innocently remarked to his mother the same night when he was being bathed that Joshua and Archibald were 'a lot bigger than he was'. On request he related the full incident and his mother had been shocked and furious, telling him that his cousins were dirty and wicked for showing themselves to him, and that their 'worms' ought to be 'cut off' if they behaved so dirtily in the future.

He had felt no disgust at their behaviour, and deduced from what his mother said to him, that he also must be 'dirty-minded' as he had not objected to their conduct.

As a teenager and young adult Henry had felt fearful and anxious, often for no reason he could define; and on the one occasion he had tried to have sex with a girl from University he had been impotent. This worried him a great deal, and made him nervous when plucking up the courage to ask a girl to go out with him. He had had a series of typical anxiety attacks, the first being precipitated by a film he watched on television, in which a corpse was discovered months after burial, covered with maggots and worms.

'I felt dreadful when I saw it,' Henry told me, 'I remembered what mother had said about "worms" being "cut off" from wicked people, and I dreamed that night that I was covered with long pink worms from my waist downward, and that mother was trying to cut them off with her gardening shears. I woke up covered in a cold sweat. I suppose I should have come to consult you then; but nothing had happened to embarrass me up to that point, although I knew I felt sick if the word "worm" was mentioned, so I left the matter well alone.'

He now acknowledged that he had a phobia towards earthworms, and accepted my explanation of how it had come into being — i.e., due to the sexual fear his mother had imbued him with at the time of his walk with his cousins, and his reaction of dread subsequently at the sight or sound of the word 'worms'.

We started therapy with some relaxation sessions, to get Henry used to the feeling of being utterly free from tension and concern and worry — which turned out to be a new experience for him, as I supposed it would. My object, then, was to accustom him to earthworms in very small degrees, until the sight of one occasioned him no bother at all.

I started by putting him into a state of medium depth trance, and describing to him in a light-hearted manner, a Children's Hour story I had seen on TV about a character named Ernie the Earthworm. He managed to listen to that with only a minimum response of tension. I told him a similar tale the following week about Ernie — this time with no tension response at all. During the next four sessions I gradually made my suggestions more and more life-like — until under deep hypnosis he was at my suggestion, actually handling an earthworm — picking it up off the path, and placing it on a patch of clean soil.

I achieved this mainly by appealing to his instincts of compassion, i.e., by suggesting that the earthworm was a small, defenceless and *harmless* creature, which deserved a modicum of help from us, on account of the good it did to the soil and the ease with which it perished if we were not kind to it. In the end I believe he was almost sorry for those earthworms! He certainly managed to 'pick one up' without any bother on the fifth occasion he came to see me. And I suggested to him that he would be relaxed in his attitude to sex as there would never be occasion for him to fear sexuality again now we had isolated the reason for his reactions.

The result of therapy was that Henry could with ease handle an earthworm without a panic attack — and had managed to raise and sustain an erection during pleasurable foreplay with his fiancée Isabelle, to whom he related the entire story. I taught him autohypnosis as a final measure, in case he found that he encountered scenes that made him nervous and phobic again. But last time I met him, he had never had to put the method into practice.

A Case of Externalization

I said that the third way the mind has of coping with unconscious anxiety, besides the production of bodily symptoms and phobias, was by externalization and identification; but one does not often get cases like this to treat, chiefly because people who unconsciously use this method, are fairly satisfied with life anyway because they help other people and see them benefit as a result.

We had one such lady patient, however, who exactly fitted the bill; her name was Consuela H. and she was English, not Spanish, which just shows that she had rather odd parents, thinking of such a name for her. She had been a nun in an enclosed Order, and came to us on the advice of her priest, who was a worldly man with a knowledge of human nature, and capable of recognizing when one of his flock needed temporal rather than purely spiritual succour. Consuela was, naturally, terrified of sex, and seemed to consider it evil even within marriage, if it were enjoyed; it seemed to her, something women had to tolerate and men had to perform in order to ensure the continuation of the human race, certainly not something to enjoy. Her parents were medical missionaries, and she had spent all her early life in a convent, while they went off to the wilds to convert pagans to Christianity.

The nuns had little trouble in convincing the impressionable eighteen-year-old girl that she had a vocation for the religious life, and six months later she entered the Noviciate with a view to becoming a nun in that Order.

During her six months of education in the outside world, however, she had undergone some interesting changes. She had studied English education at night college and had met a boy who was very attracted to her. She had repelled his advances but had liked him and could not forget him. Now back in the convent, she pursued the works of mercy with such diligence, often sitting up half the night to answer letters from foreign parts appealing for aid, that she was making herself ill, and a number of other nuns were rather upset by her zeal. The Reverend Mother had asked her time and again to contain herself — but this she was unable to do, for her worries, longings, and guilt feelings about sexuality were being sublimated in 'good works' for less fortunate people, in whose problems she buried herself wholeheartedly. However, I was asked to look into her stability (of course with her knowledge and agreement), and I deduced what I have just said. My advice to her was to have a year away from the convent, to follow whatever path presented itself, and to see where it lead her. This was met with great opposition from Consuela, but firm support from her Reverend Mother who was, in fact, a practical and likeable woman. She asked me to look after Consuela during her year of decisions.

She came to me about fifteen times in all — and I suggested to her that her mind was clear and that she felt relaxed. We discussed men and sex and love at great length — and I soon became of the opinion, that of the people innately suited to convent life Consuela was not one of them. I suggested to her, that in her fervid devotion to the problems of others, she may in fact be hiding from the real truth of herself as a desirable and lovable woman. She objected to this, very much at first; but later admitted, with many tears, that I may be right.

Over several sessions I suggested to her that the act of procreation was good and ordained by God and should therefore be enjoyed; a point she ultimately accepted. Finally she decided that lay teaching was more her vocation than an enclosed religious order and set about pursuing a teachers' training course at which she was very successful. In the end, she married a theology student and was very contented when I last heard from her, with a full time teaching career, a stable marriage and two young daughters.

10. Hypnotherapy in Practice

Apart from specific psychological conditions which can generally be traced back to childhood conflicts, a large part of a hypnotherapist's work consists of helping his patients to overcome unwanted habits. It is this kind of work for which hypnotherapists are best known, despite the fact that they also treat neurotic illnesses and personality disorders. Few of these habits are the result of identifiable trauma experienced earlier during the patient's life; the wish to keep to a slimming diet, to stop smoking or biting one's nails, or to avoid becoming flustered during an interview or driving test rarely requires deep analysis. And provided the patient feels, and appears, mentally healthy in other respects, the problem is taken at face value.

Let's look at the very common problem of ceasing to smoke. Every smoker who seeks treatment, has a different story to tell, and his or her own special difficulties with respect to doing without nicotine. Sometimes chemical addiction is the basis of recurrent failure, despite the fact that the smoker wishes sincerely to give up the habit. Occasionally, resentment at the thought of foregoing the pleasure of smoking, is the root of the problem — and when this is coupled with chemical craving for nicotine, repeated failures are hardly surprising.

We will pretend that you, the reader, are considering a course of hypnotherapy to help you to stop smoking. One of the first questions a good hypnotherapist is likely to ask you is whether you really want to relinquish this habit! You may think this is an odd question since the answer should be self-evident, but without sufficient motivation to achieve your end, you would be wasting the therapist's time and your money. As we mentioned earlier, the hypnotherapist no longer has a magic wand to wave. He can make useful suggestions to your subconscious mind which will reinforce your own will-power and help enormously if you really wish to overcome the urge to smoke. But he cannot overcome an inbuilt resistance to his suggestions. Only you know whether you really want to succeed. A few people claim that hypnotherapy has not helped them at all in their efforts to give up; but you have to ask yourself how deeply they truly wished to stop smoking in the first place.

Aversion Therapy
There are several different techniques commonly used by hypnotherapists to help patients quit the smoking habit; one is the aversion approach, in which you would first be placed in a state of light to medium trance and then be given the suggestion that cigarettes taste and smell of a substance to which you have a particular aversion. This may be old socks, cod liver oil, cow dung, the contents of a sink waste disposal unit — everyone of us can think of something that strikes us as particularly revolting! This is what the therapist using this technique would choose to liken future cigarettes to, should you think of smoking thereafter.

For some people the aversion technique works very well. They are generally people with an active imagination and a highly retentive subconscious mind which throws up the unpleasant images associated with smoking, time after time until finally the desire to smoke ceases. Some very sensitive individuals will react so strongly to the suggestions that the sight, smell and taste of cigarettes will cause them to feel — or even be — sick. But for others, the technique is less successful as the effects wear off after a couple of weeks.

'Q Day' Method
A popular and effective alternative to it is the 'Q day' method. It is less drastic and expects less of the patient, who is allowed to stop smoking gradually rather than being expected to give up the habit after a single session. If your hypnotherapist favours this approach, then the following programme or a slight variation of it is what you can expect to take place.

You will have assured the therapist that you are in earnest about wishing to stop smoking — for good. And he will doubtless ask you whether there are any special circumstances in which you find the urge to smoke irresistible, or any factors in your life which make you unduly stressed and tense. He will then be able to pay particular attention to your own personal difficulties, by including in each hypnotic session suggestions aimed at diminishing your tense feelings and enabling you better to cope with circumstances you find difficult. At the same time he will suggest to your subconscious mind, that as you grow less tense and better able to cope, so your reliance upon smoking will correspondingly diminish.

During the first visit, the hypnotherapist will map out a plan for you to follow along these lines. First you will be asked to change your brand of cigarettes — preferably to one you are not over-keen on! You will not be allowed to smoke on getting up in the morning, nor for one hour after meals, nor before going to bed at night — and you will be expected to cut down your usual daily consumption by fifty per cent. You will be instructed to hold your cigarette in the opposite hand to the one you normally use, and to help put you off cigarettes anyway, you may also be instructed to sniff hard at an ashtray of stale butt ends once or twice daily (thus incorporating an element of aversion therapy into your programme).

Follow these instructions to the letter, omitting nothing, and do not give yourself a day or two of grace before actually putting them into practice; you are faced with a difficult task and it is important that you are successful from the earliest stages of the plan. In addition, help yourself by reading anything positive on the subject of nicotine addiction that you can find. Health therapists generally emphasize the importance of a wholefood diet as a definite aid in overcoming any kind of addiction as well as setting the scene for a new and healthier lifestyle. So take advice about vitamins and find out which supplements would be of most use to you — usually L-glutamine, available from Health Food Stores, and vitamin B$_3$, dolomite and L-tryptophan are considered to be the best in combatting nicotine craving.

Since autohypnosis plays an important part in overcoming an unwanted habit, your hypnotic trance may well be induced by getting you to visualize a scene such as a garden, lake or seashore which you find particularly peaceful to contemplate. As you start to relax and picture the scene of yourself, the therapist will ask you also to picture ten steps leading down to your chosen place, down which he will ask you to walk in your imagination as he suggests to you that in so doing, you are entering more and more deeply into hypnotic trance. This will prove an invaluable aid to you at home when you practise auto-trance induction after the third session.

When you are in a state of trance, during your first visit, the suggestions likely to be made to you will be that cigarettes are a form of poison, that this poison will damage your lungs, that you absolutely rely upon healthy lungs in order to live, and that for this reason, you certainly do not need a substance which destroys them. You will also be given a graphic description of a pair of smoker's lungs, followed by one of clean healthy lungs, and reminded that while smoking causes shortness of breath, diseased arteries, an increased risk of strokes and heart attacks and cancer, these are not associated with non-smoking.

Finally when out of your trance, the therapist will very probably ask you to give yourself pre-sleep suggestions, repeating as you fall asleep: 'My desire to smoke is growing less and less', while visualizing firstly some diseased lungs and then healthy ones. And he may well suggest in addition, that you keep your cigarettes forthwith in a box clearly marked POISON!

This is not an attempt to frighten you, nor is it an example of hysterical 'overkill'; cigarette smoking is, literally, a lethal habit directly causing thousands of unnecessary deaths every month. It is also a very difficult habit to relinquish, and no-one is more aware of that fact than the hypnotherapist, except of course the smoker him or herself. That is why every gun in the therapist's armamentarium is brought to bear, when helping would-be non-smokers.

Your next appointment, usually one week after the first, is very important for it is then that 'Q day' (i.e., quitting day) is set; this is, as a rule, on the day following the third visit. During your second session, a check will be made upon your progress, and you will be asked to change your cigarette brand again; you will also be asked to cut your daily number of cigarettes by a further fifty per cent. Previous suggestions will be reinforced, together with what is known as 'ego-boosting'. This is a means of bolstering your self-confidence by emphasizing your success so far, and reinforcing your conviction of your own ability to stop smoking altogether, with the aid of the therapist. Your strong points are stressed and fears and doubts are reduced to size, and your subconscious mind starts really to believe in your ability to achieve what you wish to achieve.

You will also be taught the art of physical relaxation and asked to practise this once every day and every evening before retiring, during the forthcoming week. While doing so you will be requested to visualize the diseased and then the healthy pairs of lungs as before, while suggesting to yourself that your ability to relax in the face of stressful situations is becoming better and better, while your craving for cigarettes is growing less and less.

At the third visit your progress is again checked, as is your success in relaxing physically. You will be taught how to carry out autohypnosis, and encouraged to carry this out during the actual session so that the therapist is certain that you know how to do it. You will also — most important! - be shown how to bring yourself out of a state of self-induced hypnotic trance (usually by counting back from ten to one or zero) and the suggestion will be made to you that should an emergency arise while you are performing autohypnosis, your conscious mind will take over instantly and you will be able to cope with it.

Your therapist will ask you to use your autohypnosis sessions to suggest to yourself that from now on you will be totally free from the poisonous effects of nicotine, coal tar and the other ingredients of cigarette smoke, and that your desire for cigarettes will very rapidly become a thing of the past. You will probably be expected to go into autohypnosis once every day during the day and once again when you are about to fall asleep for the night — the only difference between the two sessions being that you do not need to count yourself back up to a fully conscious state at the end of the second session; just remain where you are, in a deeply relaxed and tranquil state and drift gently off to sleep! Your hypnosis session during your third visit will be used to reinforce all the usual helpful suggestions made during the previous two sessions, and your success to date will be emphasized, together with further ego boosting.

It will be suggested to you that you will not continue to have the slightest hankering after cigarettes, and that the excellent progress you have made to date means that your vital 'two year period' is about to commence, i.e., the two years following your last cigarette, during which the cells of your lungs regenerate healthy cells and become in fact the healthy tissue cells of lungs belonging to a non-smoker. The chance of a new 'lease of life' is stressed, and the very obvious advantages of this benefit, spelled out to your subconscious mind.

Your hypnotherapist may also mention to you that any cough

from which you may suffer is likely to grow noticeably worse for a month or two after giving up smoking! If you are warned about this in advance then it will not come as a nasty shock. The little hairs called cilia which line your wind pipe (or trachea) and the two tubes into which it divides (the right and left bronchus, one to each lung), are paralysed by cigarette smoke and are unable to perform their task of sweeping a current of mucus upwards, thus removing any foreign debris, bacteria etc. which you may inhale.

When you cease to smoke, the cilia regain their powerful action, and come to life again, removing clogged mucus, dirt, smoke debris, damaged lung cells etc. So, for about two months, you will probably have a productive cough and a certain amount of lung irritation. After that, provided that your lungs have not as yet been seriously damaged by smoking, all should be well.

The fourth session with your hypnotherapist is usually the last one. Any problems that have arisen, or episodes of backsliding, are checked, as are your continuing ability and willingness to practise total physical relaxation and autohypnosis. Finally, hypnotic suggestions are made to give a great boost to those previously made, and your success made much of.

You will probably feel great elation at your successful pursuit of your hypnotherapy course; and your therapist will certainly be similarly delighted.

Two Case Histories
Here are two short case histories of patients who have come to us for help in giving up smoking — the first to be related was initially unsuccessful while the second was an immediate success. It is interesting to give examples of failures as well as successes, but the 'one of each type' given here does not represent the ratio experienced in a normal hypnotherapy practice; successes generally outnumber failures by a factor of four to one, that is, hypnotherapy successfully helps about eighty per cent of serious would-be non-smokers to quit the habit for good.

John Lloyd sought help with his smoking problem when his attack of bronchitis lasted for longer than it should and the manager of the local football club for which he played, strongly recommended that he give up his twenty-five daily cigarettes. He had no particular emotional problems in his life nor was he a person especially subject to stress and tension. He expressed a ready willingness to give up his smoking habit in view of the present circumstances, although he admitted that he had never taken the cancer 'stories' too seriously in the past and had never tried to give up cigarettes before.

John was anxious to get the business over and done with at the earliest possible opportunity and was less keen on the 'Q day' idea than the majority of people are when told about it. He was certain that he needed only a little help in relinquishing the smoking habit, despite the fact that he had smoked every day of his life for eleven years. So the aversion method was tried.

The most revolting thing John could think of, was the smell and taste of stale, overcooked cabbage, so we likened future experiences with cigarette smoking to this, telling him that the very sight of a 'fag' as he always called them, would make him feel queasy while the taste and smell if he attempted to smoke one would make him feel too nauseous to continue — so redolent would it be of the vegetable he loathed.

He went away promising to let us know — but absolutely certain in his own mind of success. Consciously, that is. Regrettably, his subconscious mind failed to retain the acuteness of the initial image which worked so well for him for the first three or four days; and the next after-match drinking session saw him light up several cigarettes in the company of his friends, without too much interference from subconscious aversive images.

John was back on the Monday morning following the Saturday night failure, honest in admitting that he had underestimated the size of the problem and ready to try the method we prefer, of working steadily towards a 'Q day' goal. He was a model patient and although still impatient to reach success, he persisted with the techniques we instructed him in, finding to his surprise a great propensity and liking for auto-hypnosis and physical relaxation sessions. He reached 'Q day' without any undue problems and telephoned three months later of his own accord to assure us of his continuing success. I think his particular motivation to let us know all was well, was an understandable few moments of euphoria after he had scored a record number of match goals!

Sue Jennings, an attractive thirty-year-old secretary, decided to stop smoking for two reasons; her mother had just undergone an operation to remove a large section of her left lung, which was found to be cancerous — she, the mother, aged fifty-six, had smoked between thirty and forty cigarettes every day of her life since the age of fifteen. And Sue, married for five years and wanting to start a family, had just discovered that she was at last pregnant.

She had no particular nervous or emotional problems, apart from the fact that she disliked her boss's partner and had to spend one day per week in his company while her own particular boss visited Head Office for a weekly Sales Conference. This particular man was sarcastic and bad tempered, and insisted on dictating at a speed far beyond the shorthand capacity of the vast majority of efficient shorthand typists. Consequently, every Friday was a time of great stress for Sue, and her cigarette consumption reflected this fact, increasing to as many as forty on that day of the week as opposed to fifteen to twenty on other days.

So we dealt first with this problem, and I gave her sufficient ego boosting to allow her to face Fridays with a certain amount of calm assurance; she was even able to stand up for herself when Mr Peters was particularly scathing, and as success generally breeds success, not only did her confidence in herself grow from strength to strength but he himself took stock of the situation and actually became less of a bully. Success in this respect did not come overnight and there were one or two setbacks; but three sessions were sufficient to cope with this particular problem.

I decided, with Sue's full agreement, to cope separately with her fears and lack of confidence as, apart from the smoking problem, she was also experiencing regular weekend migraine attacks. Having got the stress factors in her life under control, we embarked upon a further four sessions employing the 'Q day' technique. So pleased was Sue at her increased ability to cope at work and the cessation of her migraine attacks, that she followed all my instructions to the letter and was eager and ready for 'Q day' when it arrived.

She had proved a naturally good hypnotic subject and had practised autohypnosis coupled with autosuggestion twice daily as I had asked her to — unlike John Lloyd who had admitted to forgetting to do so once or twice until he became convinced of the necessity for it. So the net gain of a total of seven sessions of hypnotherapy to Sue Jennings was considerably greater self-confidence, no further migraine attacks, happier working conditions, and success in efforts to stop smoking.

Weight Control

I have dealt with smoking in relation to the practice of hypnotherapy in considerable detail, because it constitutes one of the commonest problems with which hypnotherapists are asked to deal. But we should also look at some of the other frequent reasons, apart from psychological disturbances, which prompt people to seek this type of therapy.

Weight control is one of these. Because of the associations we have all to a certain extent learned to make, between a slim, lithe figure, sexual attractiveness and personal happiness, feelings on this subject run very deep, no less among the minority of individuals who wish to gain weight than among people with the commoner problem of wishing to lose it. Understandably, there is precious little sympathy between these two groups, skinny men and women envying their 'well covered' partners, friends and family members just as much, and just as justifiably, as the fatties who long to swop places with all the thin people they know.

Apart from relatively rare instances in which malfunctioning glands are at the root of the problem, weight control is basically a matter of either eating too much or of eating far too little in relation to the metabolic rate of the particular person concerned. Doctors and hypnotherapists alike, see very many people within the course of a year's practice, who complain that although they eat as little (or conversely as much) as the normally built people around them whom they cite as examples, they themselves fail completely to lose, or to gain, an ounce.

When this is true, and they are neither 'forgetting' to eat, nor overlooking a number of high calorie snacks eaten between meals, the reason for their failing to alter their weight as they wish is simply that their own particular metabolisms burn fuel (i.e., food) more slowly or more quickly than those of many people around them. So a fat person, for example, would still be taking in too many calories for his personal requirements, despite the fact that he had reduced his calorie intake to, say, one thousand calories per day.

With many of us, therefore, being overweight is a straightforward matter of eating too much! But while the problem may be easy to solve theoretically — dieting is in no way an easy task, any more than is giving up the habit of smoking. If it were, there would be far fewer fat men and women collectively spending millions of pounds every year in failed attempts to lose weight.

There are numerous reasons why people eat too much. Sometimes it is a matter of ignorance of the fact that they burn food fuel especially slowly and so need to cut down their daily food intake far more than, say, another obese person with an ordinarily functioning metabolism whose main problem is a love of sweets and chocolate. Hypnotherapy can help enormously with weight problems — but just as I pointed out in connection with the smoking habit, the most highly skilled therapist in the world is useless unless the patient really wishes to lose weight and maintain a new, low one. There is no magic wand available to be waved, and a great deal of effort is required on behalf of the subject.

Eating binges can form part of an obsessive illness, just as persistent nibbling can be an aspect of obsessive or compulsive tendencies. As is so often true, the dividing line between 'normal' and 'abnormal' is a very fine one, and possibly there are elements of obsessive-compulsive behaviour in all abnormal eating patterns. But as I pointed out at the beginning of the present chapter, thousands of ordinary people seek hypnotherapy to help them to slim, stop smoking etc. without there being any underlying psychological abnormality whatsoever. Ann Bowen was a typical example, and these were her circumstances.

She was a pleasant, intelligent woman of thirty-five, who had put on too much weight during her two pregnancies and had failed to lose any since. For several years she had told herself that plumpness was nothing to worry about, but for the past eighteen months she had weighed over twelve stone and had tried unsuccessfully to slim. She had cut her calorie intake to nine hundred per day, and had lost a few pounds each time she had done so — only to regain them immediately she tried to eat normally for a couple of days to relieve the boredom. She was also a nibbler!

'Unfortunately I adore chocolate,' she confessed. 'At one time it didn't bother me; but ever since Tim, my husband, started to go out alone in the evening, I've been stocking up on Mars bars to eat in front of the TV once I've put the children to bed; last night I actually got through five of them!'

I thought that this may well be a vicious circle, with her husband typically losing interest in his overweight wife, who in turn began to rely on the very foods that were increasing her problem, by way of compensation. So I told Ann that successful weight reduction would never be one of her achievements unless she altered her eating patterns permanently — and gave her a diet to follow that contained as many of her favourite food items as possible while eliminating all junk food, white sugar, sweetmeats and between-meal carbohydrate snacks.

She came for hypnotherapy on a weekly basis, over a seven month period — which is considerably longer than many hypnotherapists would expect a patient to continue coming. I find, however, that while weight is quite easily lost with the aid of hypnotic suggestion, many patients fall by the wayside when no longer attending for therapy. Psychological, or emotional, dependence upon fattening foods is a difficult bond to sever completely, and until food is no longer thought of as a substitute for love, stress, the occasional row with a marital partner, and sometimes simple boredom, can tip the scales, in both senses of the expression, against the patient's chances of lasting slimness.

Many overweight people have tried and failed so many times to lose weight that they are often practically in despair about the matter. Belief in the possibility of success is an important element in effective hypnotherapy, so I impressed upon Ann that she was perfectly capable of achieving a slim figure if she would play her part in our mutual effort — which she was very willing to do once she was convinced that there was a chance of victory.

Then I set out, as I do with all obese patients, to help Ann to change her eating habits. I began with some suggestions to boost her ego and reinforce her self-confidence; and followed this by implanting the idea that every day she would grow more and more relaxed and calm, and that this in turn would lead to a greater measure of self-confidence and improved self-control.

This, I suggested to her subconscious mind, would bring about a condition in which she derived greater pleasure from low-calorie foods than she had ever done before, and that as salads, fruit, vegetables and lean meat grew increasingly appealing, so she would lose her desire for fattening foods. I told her that every day, her wish and determination to stick to her diet would grow more and more strong, until eventually her craving for frankly fattening foods would cease altogether.

Every time Ann came for a treatment session I would weigh her, chart her weight loss on her own personal weight loss graph, and discuss any particular problems she was having. Despite one or two disappointing weeks in which she gained a couple of pounds — generally consequent upon a weighing-in session which showed less weight loss than she would have liked to see — the course was completely successful and she achieved her target of eight stone, which was ideal for her height and build and the weight she had maintained all her adult life prior to her first pregnancy.

Marjorie Diggins was a nineteen-year-old model, who worked under the name of Jolie Monet and who had, so her agent told her, great potential in her chosen field, provided she could manage by some means or another, to enlarge her bustline. Marjorie was a tiny size-eight, tall, and with skin, hair and facial features to be proud of — but her bust measurement was slightly less than thirty-two inches. This would probably have been ideal a decade or so ago, when Twiggy figures were the most dearly prized, but nowadays photographers and fashion magazines prefer their models to look rather better nourished, at least with respect to their having rounded breasts, and Marjorie was desperate to find a way of solving her problem.

Models have the same figure problems as the rest of womankind when it comes to regional control; and she discovered that if she deliberately ate more than usual, her weight would increase to the disadvantage of her hip measurements and leave her tiny breasts completely unchanged. Exercises had had no effect, and she was considering the drastic remedy of expensive plastic surgery when a friend of hers suggested she try hypnotherapy. Hence her appointment with us.

It is not very commonly known that bustlines can be improved by hypnotic suggestion, but the fact remains that they can and often are — provided, as always, that the woman has the prerequisite amount of patience and a strong desire for the goal to be achieved.

The case of Peta Smythe should be mentioned here in passing; she was brought for bust enlargement therapy by her rich fiancé, and there was no response whatsoever to the suggestions that her bustline would increase. We gently probed the matter further and it transpired that Peta, a naturally timid girl, hadn't the slightest desire for larger breasts and was perfectly contented with the size she was. It was simply a wish to please her fiancé that had brought her to us, and the net result of ego boosting, was not the necessity for a larger bra size but the ditching of her rather overbearing fiancé in preference for the man she really wanted to marry — who loved her exactly the way she was!

I mentioned Peta's story to Marjorie to impress upon her that a real wish to succeed was essential; but she was so strongly motivated towards a successful modelling career that she could barely wait for the sessions to commence!

Briefly, besides the usual ego boosting, I regressed Marjorie to the age of twelve, which was when she could remember the feeling and the sensation of her breasts enlarging. I got her to experience this phase of development as vividly as possible, and taught her relaxation and autohypnosis so that she could induce the same feeling at home on a daily or twice-daily basis. I also asked her to imagine that her breasts were growing to the desired size, and to retain this image in her mind during her autohypnotic sessions whilst she was reproducing the actual physical sensations associated with their early development.

Marjorie practised the technique assiduously, and after attending for hypnotherapy once a week for three months, her bustline had increased by two and a half inches. Career success came soon afterwards and she was delighted to tell us, a month later, that she had been commissioned to model a collection of winter knitwear for a leading women's magazine.

Nail Biting

Nail biting is a very common problem and can be a simple habit acquired during childhood in response to transitory feelings of insecurity, or part of a more complex pattern of anxiety neurosis or obsessive compulsive behaviour. When small children bite their nails, it is usually the parents who worry about the habit and not the child; and it generally either reflects the desire to combat the dominating attitude of a parent or represents simple oral comfort following an anxiety-generating event.

Christina Martin, aged eight, was brought to us by her mother, who reported that her daughter's nail biting habit had started six months earlier following the birth of a sibling. Mrs Martin admitted that her baby son took up a great deal of her time and energy, but had tried to compensate by showing Christina as much love as possible. Christina had settled down in other respects and was beginning to accept the presence of a baby brother — but continued to bite her nails almost incessantly.

She was a well-adjusted child in other respects and there was no real reason to suspect the existence of a deep seated psychological problem. I told her during our first session together, that she was a pretty little girl and would be even prettier with nicely shaped fingernails. I asked her to confine her chewing to a finger on each hand selected by herself (the index finger in each case) and suggested to her under hypnosis that she would from that time onwards, wish to become as pretty as possible in every way — thereby losing the wish to bite her nails to the quick.

She managed to bite only the two chosen fingers by the time she came for her third appointment, and I told her she would soon have every reason to feel proud of her hands. I also employed the aversion approach to telling her that she would experience a very bitter taste every time she put her fingers in her mouth and that this would make her feel sick if she persisted in chewing her nails.

Christina came for a total of four treatment sessions and she did lose her nail biting habit; she did pick at her nails for a time but I was able to suggest to her that this was a great pity as it would undo all her great efforts in ceasing to bite them. By this time they were longer and her mother had even been able to manicure them for her. I suggested to Mrs Martin that she buy her little girl an inexpensive manicure set of her own and also a cheap bottle of clear nail varnish.

This worked admirably, and meeting them both in the High Street three months after the last appointment, I was greeted with the information that Christina liked long nails so much nowadays, especially when she was allowed to paint them, that the only remaining problem was persuading her to cut or file them!

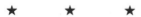

Finally, in attempting to sum up various aspects of the healing power of hypnotism, we will take a quick reminding glance at the illnesses which can be helped and often cured by the practice of this therapy — and re-emphasize those not normally treated by any of its methods.

Hypnotherapy can help people suffering from compulsive behaviour, depression and a schizoid personality. These are abnormalities deriving from unresolved conflict at the oral stage of development and generally respond well to hypnosis. One word should be said about depressive illness. I mentioned earlier that hypnotherapy was useful to people suffering from mild to moderate depression; this is so, but in the case of an individual who is severely ill with depressive symptoms, and in an inert, non-functional condition with, perhaps, suicidal tendencies — the place for his immediate treatment is a hospital, either as an In-Patient, or on a 'daily visit' basis; or, at the very least, at home in bed where he is being taken care for.

All these settings are appropriate ones for the administration of first line treatment of choice in the severely depressed patient, which is drug therapy. This is *not* to advocate the view that depression should really be treated by drugs and drugs alone; the longterm administration of neither tricyclic nor MAOI anti-depressants, is in any sense the ideal approach, nor does it ever seem to cure patients.

But the fact remains, that a man or woman with severe depression is a very sick individual, and because of his or her degree of mental torpor and withdrawal, is in no condition *initially* to reap benefit from either hypno-analysis or hypnotherapy. The role of anti-depressant drugs, is to combat the incapacating symptoms of the illness, by raising the patient's subjective feelings and lightening his mood. This will place him in a position in which he will be capable of communicating, albeit poorly at first, with his therapist, and of responding to hypnotherapeutic measures.

Next, hypnotherapy can relieve people suffering from 'anal phase' abnormalities such as obsessive behaviour and hypochondria; it is not used in paranoid individuals who are subject to delusions and illusions, and who may be made worse by the treatment. The fact that one of Freud's reasons for abandoning hypnosis as a therapeutic method, was its failure to provide a permanent cure for hysterical illness, should be born in mind, as should his failure to plant a permanent and lasting post-hypnotic suggestion. However, another of his objections to hypnosis was the fact that he could not induce really deep hypnotic trances in his subjects, so it is possible that these three facts are closely interrelated and the first, the result of the other two.

But in the treatment of obsessive habits and thought patterns, and in the elimination of hypochondriacal symptoms, hypnotherapy skilfully used can work wonders. And the word 'wonders' takes us all the way back to the history of the use of trance, and the 'miracle cures' which in olden times were attributed to the benevolence of the gods. There is nothing really either 'wondrous' or 'miraculous' about the cures that hypnosis can produce; but when numerous other traditional methods of medicine, surgery and/or pharmaceuticals have been applied to a problem without success, then a cure effected by means of trance induction and hypnotic suggestion can certainly seem wondrous — both to the patient, and to those who live with/care for him.

Thirdly, the neuroses resulting from genital phase conflicts — hysteria and anxiety state, usually respond well to hypnotherapy. The use of abreaction can be especially useful in treating the former, especially when painful events in the patient's life history *can* be tied up with the development of conversion symptoms. Reliving (revivifying) the painful occasion often dramatically dispels the most florid of symptoms — once, of course, the patient is motivated to their removal himself.

Hypnotherapy is not as a rule used for epileptic patients — and it is safe to say 'never used' in patients who are categorized as 'insane'. These constitute a large group of mentally sick people with a variety of illnesses, the different forms of schizophrenia being the best known, and the 'group word' for which is the 'psychoses'.

People suffering from psychotic illness differ from those affected by neurotic illness, in that they are out of touch with reality. Neurosis does not affect normal reasoning and whatever the degree of emotional disturbance the conscious mind keeps a grip upon reality, retaining its ability to distinguish between fact and fiction and not becoming the subject of delusions, illusions or hallucinations. The neurotic patient is fully aware of his disorder although he may be unable to identify it; the psychotic is unaware of his, due to the fact that he cannot distinguish fact from fiction.

Psychotic illness may be either due to an organic disturbance, in which the brain cells are damaged in some way, for example by alcohol, drugs and poisons or injury; or to a functional disturbance, in which the mind and thought processes are disturbed without any signs of physical disease. Schizophrenia is one of the two major functional psychotic illnesses — and the other is manic-depressive psychosis, a severe form of depression in which bouts of depressive illness alternate with bouts of abnormal euphoria and hyperactivity, called mania.

Appendix
Theories of Hypnosis
and Some Proven Applications

Definitions of the mechanism of hypnosis abound and are constantly being revised and expanded as further research continues. Nearly all theories add something to our knowledge of the subject whilst none can be considered totally conclusive. Consequently it may be instructive to run through some of the more important theories in order to arrive at a reasonably satisfactory definition of the trance state and its mechanisms.

Interestingly enough, hypnosis itself was at one time thought to be the symptom of a neurosis! The eminent French psychologist, Charcot, who did so much to further the cause of the therapeutic use of hypnotism, believed that only hysterical patients could be hypnotized. However, though hysterics are perhaps as a group more easily hypnotizable that is not to say that the easily hypnotizable person is an hysteric!

Another interesting theory is linked with the study of animal hypnosis. This considers the hypnotic trance to be comparable to the immobility reflex which causes an animal to freeze when in danger and thereby escape notice. Both humans and animals do share this reflex when presented with a powerful stimulus such as fear. But there the similarity would appear to end; animals respond to physical and instinctual constraints whilst humans respond not just to these but also to the interaction of words, symbols and meanings.

Hypnosis and Sleep
The actual word 'hypnosis' derives from a Greek word, 'hypnos' meaning sleep and was coined by the Scottish physician James Braid in 1842. Pavlov in 1957 stated that hypnosis was a 'partial sleep' since both hypnosis and sleep create inhibition in some areas of the brain. Other researchers believe that the trance state is a

modified form of sleep. The basis of the 'sleep' theories is the fact that relaxation is brought about by the rhythmic and monotonous repetition of stimuli whilst the narrowing of the focus of attention creates immobilization and inhibits some mental functions. However, this theory is not tenable since it has been shown that the two states are physiologically different.

There is no loss of consciousness during hypnosis and reflex actions such as the knee jerk still function whereas during sleep both are lost. Other studies such as investigations into blood pressure and physiochemical activity together with the monitoring of brain activity by EEG apparatus indicate that hypnosis is neither a true sleeping state nor a true waking state. Russian researchers in particular have demonstrated that there are definite changes in both the physical and psychological states of a subject when in hypnosis. They concluded that hypnosis is a special state that exists in its own right.

Additionally Pavlov believed that hypnosis is related to conditioning and therefore is a reaction linked with past experience. Words, like experience, can act as a stimuli and produce physical and psychological responses. There is, of course, a considerable amount of truth in this, since the hypnotist, during the induction stage, endeavours to induce conditioned responses to his words and intonation. However, this can only be a part of the mechanism of hypnosis — not the complete answer.

The Psychoanalytic Theory

The psychoanalytic theory has many staunch supporters[3] and is based, in the main, on the concept of regression to childhood with the subject viewing the hypnotist in the role of parent. Consequently the love, respect and fear that the subject felt as a child for a particular parent is transferred to the hypnotist with the result that the subject then wishes to obey him. The hypnotist is then free to remould the regressed state in order to produce the beneficial results required by the subject. Gill and Brenman, for instance, consider that hypnosis is a 'regression in the service of the ego' and that the transference referred to above is a very important part of the mechanism.

There is no doubt that transference often does play a vital role in hypnosis and can sometimes lead to attachment to the therapist which has to be handled very carefully. It was this aspect of hypnosis which caused Freud considerable embarrassment when a patient threw her arms round him after coming out of trance! However, such extreme behaviour is fortunately rare. Regression and transference may play an important part in the hypnotic process for some subjects but not for all; moreover such a theory cannot account for the ability of most people to utilize autohypnosis (self-hypnosis).

Dissociation

The dissociation theory which has been well supported in the past (Janet and others) maintained that a hypnotized person was in a dissociated state in which certain areas of behaviour and activity were separated out from the mainstream of awareness with the result that the subject lost volition and reacted in an automatic fashion. Thus the conscious mind is considered to have dissociated and another part of the subject's mind is regarded as replacing it. Few nowadays subscribe to this theory.

Role-Playing

Some psychologists consider that hypnosis is nothing more or less than role-playing on the part of the subject and that the hypnotized person behaves according to his own expectation of how a hypnotized person should behave. Obviously a subject who comes to a hypnotherapist often has preconceived ideas about hypnotism and the hypnotic trance but it is part of the therapist's job to enlighten the subject about hypnotism, give any necessary explanations and tell him what to expect.

Even so, because of the rapport that must necessarily develop between the therapist and his patient and the patient's motivation to get well and co-operate with the therapist, it is very likely that there is some degree of role playing in the early stages of the therapeutic relationship. This, however, is far from providing a satisfactory theory since it takes no account of the fact that young children can be hypnotized and they would have but little idea of the role they were expected to play. Nor can it explain controlled regression to childhood and the recovery of repressed material.

Hypersuggestibility

Some investigators, such as Barber, have propounded the theory of hypersuggestibility. They suggest that the subject's spectrum of attention is restricted to the hypnotist's voice and words resulting in the therapist taking over the subject's inner voice. This would presume that most people who can be hypnotized are hypersuggestible, which is not the case, and would also imply a fair degree of dominance on the part of the hypnotist as is indicated by the citing of mob orators and successful salesmen as a form of proof; whereas most therapists nowadays tend to avoid an authoritarian approach. This is not to say that the hypnotist does not often use a subtle form of persuasion for the subject's own good.

Altered States

The recent upsurge of interest in Yoga, Eastern techniques of meditation and modern variants such as Transcendental Meditation, together with occultism in general has encouraged many to suggest that hypnosis is basically a state of altered consciousness. Behavioural therapeutics and the use of imagery conditioning during hypnosis have further stimulated interest in this idea. Certainly, meditation over the ages has proved an effective method of behaviour modification and of goal directed striving with ultimate success. Clearly the chanting of prayers or mantras, repetition, candles, incense, a relaxed and harmonious atmosphere, posture or postural movement such as swaying, and eye fixation on an altar or a symbol are hypnogogic and contain many of the ingredients of hypnotic induction. Additionally, the seclusion, self-discipline, self-study and imaging ability required for meditation are similar to the requirements for successful auto-hypnosis.

All the methods referred to in the previous paragraph require the student to engage in conditioning ritual and most of them use the power of imaging to achieve the desired end. It is also noticeable that all methods require the reduction of external stimuli to extremely low levels. Investigation has shown that there is a common neurophysical and EEG foundation to all states of altered consciousness including that attained in the deepest form of hypnosis.

The Mind as an Electronic Device

The screening out of unwanted stimuli in hypnosis and similar states has also been compared to the elimination of interference in electronic communications systems, thus enabling a transmitter to communicate accurately with a receiver. Further comparison of the mind with computers has ensued. It has been suggested that the mind usually functions as a general purpose computer but that when in hypnosis it acts as a special purpose computer, receiving, acknowledging and acting upon only selected data. Thus the hypnotist becomes the transmitter/keyboard and the subject the receiver/computer, the essential factor being the intense concentration on the therapist's voice with the resultant abolition of interference or distortion.

How do the hypnotist's words reach the computer/mind and what happens within the computer when it receives the selective signals? Much research has been done into this question and continues to be done.

The Limbic System
The ascending reticular formation (specific part of the central nervous system) is the means by which the transmission of stimuli to the cerebral areas is affected; its involvement in hypnosis has been investigated by De Moraes Passos.[4] Assessing research into the ascending reticular formation and the brain in connection with hypnosis, Waxman considers it and the limbic area of the brain to be of paramount importance in the creation of hypnosis.[5]

The limbic area has several components and its total function is still a matter for research. However, it is known that two of its structures (the amygdala and the hypothalamus) are concerned with anxiety. The first of these is concerned with emotion and the second communicates with the cortex (the active, thinking, decision-making area of the brain) which makes feelings and emotions conscious and initiates appropriate responses. Thus external stimulus producing anger or fear first travels along the ascending reticular system to the limbic system and thence to the cortex resulting in conscious appreciation and reaction.

In a similar fashion it is thought that the hypnotist's voice travels along the reticular system and, because of the induction techniques used by the hypnotist, all other stimuli are reduced to minimal proportions thus resulting in the focussing of the subject's attention entirely on the words of the therapist. The limbic area receives the therapist's communication and passes it on to the appropriate section of the brain with the result that all emotional reactions and their concomitants are subdued and the subject enters a state of physical and psychological quiesence which equates with hypnosis.

Of all the current theories the one described in the last paragraph has, in our opinion, the most to commend it. Such a theory is able to incorporate a number of valid facts from other theories. Obviously it can include biochemical and physiological changes in the body and consequently the work of such researchers as Peters and Stern who carried out investigations into variations in blood-pressure and skin temperature during hypnotic induction[6] or Edmonston who measured the electrodermal responses during hypnosis.[7] Hypnosis as an altered state of consciousness fits in easily and so does the idea of the brain as an electronic receiver/computer.

The limbic theory, loosely designated, also explains the way in which the therapist can control the situation during hypnosis and how it is possible for him to arouse the emotions attendant upon a past traumatic event and create an abreaction when such a course of action seems desirable.

Ideas as Drugs

An interesting corollary to the above is Arthur Janov's theory that ideas can function as opiates. In his book *Prisoners of Pain** he states that: 'The best possible tranquilliser in the world is an idea. Ideas are not *like* opiates they *are* opiates. They enter the brain where they pick up meaning, become transmuted into biochemical processes . . . and end up suppressing pain.' The 'biochemical processes' are important since he believes that words/ideas can produce endorphines — naturally occurring pain-killing substances which circulate through the body to achieve their aim. One example is beta-endorphine, forty-eight times stronger than morphine, which is secreted simultaneously with the stress hormone ACTH irrespective of whether the causative factor is physical, emotional or mental, or any combination of these.

Biochemical reaction to external stimuli and the production of endorphines play a part in Janov's theory of pain and of neuroses. Here, however, the postulation of 'ideas as opiates' and their biochemical results fits in easily with what we have been discussing about the limbic system and hypnosis. Suggested ideas, thoughts, words, images in hypnosis obviously have a tranquillizing effect and can be used to alleviate or suppress pain whether psychic or physical.

* *Prisoners of Pain*, Arthur Janov, Sphere, London 1982.

Conclusion on Theories

Although it has barely been possible to do more than scratch the surface of a subject as complex as the mechanism of hypnosis, most of the theories about it contribute something useful. From the findings of many different investigators it is possible to build up a useful composite theory about hypnosis and the one described in the last few paragraphs seems to us to be reasonable. Research continues apace and no doubt new theories will arise; eventually as knowledge increases specialist investigators will finally merge and lead to a composite and definitive picture which will be accepted by the majority of practitioners.

Some Successes of Hypnotherapy

We have written a great deal about theories of hypnosis but what about its efficacy in therapeutics? Obviously, we have our own experience and that of colleagues to go on. That in itself we find convincing otherwise we would not have written this book nor be practising hypnotherapy!

The Nineteenth Century

The success story of hypnotherapy, as we know it, extends back into nineteenth century Mesmerism, as it was then known, after Anton Mesmer, whom we have already mentioned, attracted the attention of John Elliotson, the first professor of medicine at the University College Hospital. He rapidly became enthusiastic about its use and consequently fell foul of the orthodox medical establishment of the time and defiantly resigned his post. Between 1840 and 1850, James Esdale, practising in India reported some three hundred painless operations through the use of Mesmerism. In France, during the latter part of the nineteenth century, Leibault of Nancy who was later joined by Bernheim treated over 12,000 patients with a considerable amount of success. In many respects these two can be considered to have fathered the modern therapeutic applications of hypnosis.

Hypnotherapy Today

Today hypnosis has many and varied uses. In psychotherapy alone Roy Udolf in his *Handbook of Hypnosis for Professionals**

* *Handbook of Hypnosis for Professionals*, Roy Udolf, Von Nostrand Rheinhold, 1980.

lists its use in the following complaints: alcoholism, children's night terrors, conversion headache, depression, drug addiction, enuresis, hypochondriasis, frigidity, hysteria, impotence, insomnia, migraine, multiple personality, nail biting, overeating, phobias, psychogenic seizures, psychogenic tremors, psychosomatic disorders, schizophrenia, sexual disorders, smoking, speech disorders, suicidal tendencies, tics. It is an impressive list!

Smoking

The dangers of the smoking habit to health are now well known and it is not surprising therefore that many people seek help from hypnotherapists in order to conquer the addiction. Studies in the United States and elsewhere have shown a fair degree of success in the use of hypnosis for this problem. One of the highest success rates, 82 per cent, was obtained by Crasilneck and Hall. Watkins also achieved considerable success and a follow-up showed that 67 per cent of the subjects used in the study had not resumed smoking at the end of six months. Barber on the other hand claimed that after the lapse of a year the best cure rate obtainable was 20 per cent. Certainly hypnotherapy is not a magic cure for smoking but the fact remains that it can successfully help a large number of people. What is clear from studies on the problem is that strong initial motivation on the part of the person being treated is of the utmost importance.

Obesity

Obesity is another common problem for which a large number of ladies consult hypnotherapists. Here hypnosis alone will achieve little; it has to be accompanied by a planned programme of diet, exercise, relaxation and investigation of causative factors. Kroger has achieved a success rate of about 60 per cent using group therapy involving four or five patients. During the sessions his subjects are also taught auto-hypnosis as an additional aid.

Breast Enlargement

Just as many women are concerned that they have lost their figure through being overweight, others are concerned about appearing sufficiently feminine owing to the small size of their breasts. Hypnosis has been used to remedy this situation. Williams[8] in twelve sessions, at weekly intervals, caused thirteen subjects to average an increase of 2.11 inches in breast circumference. Others have followed in his footsteps with equal success and it would appear that in the majority of cases the enlargement was maintained.

Skin Problems

Dermatological problems often respond well to hypnosis, particularly the treatment of warts. It is estimated that 60 to 70 per cent of warts react to this type of therapy. Acne and other cosmetically disturbing complaints also respond well. Kroger has also obtained 'gratifying success' in the treatment of pruritus vulvae (irritation of the vaginal membranes).

Hiccups

Hiccups which are severe enough for surgical intervention to be considered have been reported to respond to treatment by hypnosis. According to Kroger, and others, approximately 75 per cent of sufferers from chronic hiccups can be helped.

Tinnitus

Tinnitus (head noises) can be a most distressing complaint from which it is difficult to obtain relief. Particularly annoying are the attacks of dizziness associated with it in many cases. Investigators have shown that the use of hypnosis can considerably alleviate the intensity and often the frequency of the noises whilst a 50 per cent success rate has been achieved in the treatment of associated dizziness.

Hypnosis and the Control of Pain

Hypnosis can be used with varying degrees of success in the relief of pain. Schafer[9] used hypnosis to alleviate pain in severely burned patients and was able to diminish pain levels in 70 per cent for the group he studied. Bachet and Weiss treated a series of patients who had suffered amputation of limbs by means of group hypnosis and attained a success rate in excess of 80 per cent[10]. Even the terrible pain of cancer has been alleviated by hypnotherapeutic measures. Kroger has treated patients in varying stages of cancer and noted that some 20 per cent could control their pain and that the need for narcotic drugs was drastically reduced among another 40 per cent.

Conclusion

There has not been space here to mention, however briefly, more than a very few of the investigations and studies relating to theories about hypnosis and the curative value that its use has in many different fields. Nor have we touched upon non-therapeutic uses such as those employed for military purposes or methods used to obtain the maximum performance from a sportsman or an athlete. Hopefully we have written sufficient to show that hypnosis has many serious applications, and that, although it is no panacea, it has considerable success in a variety of situations. Though there is as yet no single theory of hypnosis which is acceptable to all, the value of hypnosis as a therapy, both alone and in combination with other methods of treatment, is increasingly recognized.

References

1. J. P. Melei and E. R. Hilgardi: 'Attitudes towards hypnosis, self-predictions, and hypnotic susceptilibility'. *Int. J. Clin. Exp. Hyp.* 12: 99-108, 1964.

2. T. X. Barber, I. Karacan and D. S. Calverley: 'Hypnotizability and suggestibility in chronic schizophrenics'. *Arch. Gen. Psychiat.* II: 439-51, 1964.

3. Kubie, L.S., and Margolin, S.: 'The Process of Hypnotism and the Nature of the Hypnotic State'. *Am. J. Psychiat.*, 100: 613, 194.

   Gill, M.M., and Brenman, M.: *Hypnosis and Related States: Psychoanalytic Studies in Regression*. New York, International Universities Press, 1959.

4. De Moraes Passos, A.S.: 'Reflections on Hypnosis and the Reticular System of the Brain Stem'. *Hypnosis and Psychosomatic Medicine*. New York, Springer-Verlag, 1967, pp. 228-232.

5. Waxman, D.: *Hypnosis: A Guide For Patients And Practitioners*. London, George Allen and Unwin Ltd., 1981.

6. Peters, J.E. and Stern, R.M.: 'Peripheral Skin Temperature and Vasomotor Response During Hypnotic Induction'. *Int. J. Clin. Exp. Hyp.* 21:102, 1973.

7. Edmonston, W.E.: 'Hypnosis and Electrodermal Responses'. *Am. J. Clin. Hyp.* 11: 16, 1968.

8. Williams, J.E.: 'Stimulation of Breast Growth by Hypnosis'. *J. Sex Research*, 10: 316, 1974.

9. Schafer, D.W.: 'Hypnosis Use on a Burn Unit'. *Int. J. Clin. Exp. Hypn.* 23:1, 1975.

10. Bachet, M., and Weiss, C.: 'Treatment of Disorders of Amputated Subjects by Hypnotic Inhibition'. *Br. J. Med. Hyp.*, 4: 15, 1952.

Useful Addresses

The National Council of Psychotherapists and Hypnotherapy
Register*
1 Clovelly Road
Ealing
London W5

Blythe College of Hypnosis and Psychotherapy
168 Brownside Road
Worsthorne
Burnley
Lancs. BB10 3JW

The British Society of Medical and Dental Hypnosis
42 Links Road
Ashtead
Surrey KT21 2HJ

The British Society for Experimental and Clinical Hypnosis
10 Manhattan Drive
Cambridge
CB4 1JL

* The National Council of Psychotherapists provides a list of their
members practising in any given area.

Index